Simulation in Acute Neurology

Simulation in Acute Neurology

SARA E. HOCKER, MD
Associate Professor of Neurology, Mayo Clinic College of Medicine
Practice Chair, Department of Neurology, Hospital Practice
Director, Neurocritical Care Fellowship
Consultant, Neurosciences Intensive Care Unit
Mayo Clinic, Rochester, MN, United States

EELCO F. M. WIJDICKS, MD, PHD, FACP, FNCS
Professor of Neurology, Mayo Clinic College of Medicine
Chair, Division of Critical Care Neurology
Consultant, Neurosciences Intensive Care Unit
Mayo Clinic, Rochester, MN, United States

ELSEVIER

ELSEVIER

3251 Riverport Lane
St. Louis, Missouri 63043

Publisher: Mica Haley
Acquisition Editor: Melanie Tucker
Editorial Project Manager: Jennifer Horigan
Production Project Manager: Poulouse Joseph
Cover Designer: James Rownd, Alan Studholme
Typeset by TNQ Technologies

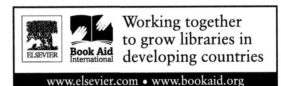

Preface

Medical training using simulation is a tested complement to the apprentice model. Simulation centers provide this teaching opportunity, and there we can also act out neurologic emergencies. This method of training is necessary because the opportunities to teach rapid-fire decisions and, thus to effectively triage acutely ill neurologic patients, is rarely present. Adequate exposure to major neurologic emergencies for physicians in training cannot be guaranteed with current curricula, and the competency of handling acute neurologic disorders—often deteriorating inconspicuously—is unknown. Many of these neuroemergencies can be reproduced in a simulation center, allowing direct observation of our trainees' clinical skills. Teachable scenarios may include recognition of imminent neuromuscular respiratory failure, recognition of a deteriorating patient with an acute brain lesion, and treatment of refractory status epilepticus. Virtually any neurologic emergency can be written in a scenario as long as the focus is on recognition and management.

Simulating Acute Neurology is a textbook on the development and execution of a simulation-based educational program in the evaluation and management of acute neurologic emergencies. *Simulating Acute Neurology* has practical value because it contains detailed descriptions of our simulation scenarios. The foundation of this book is our experience with neurosimulation, and it has been a very good one.

Part I provides an overview of the principles of simulation in medicine and examines the many unique opportunities simulation provides as an educational tool. Barriers to simulating neurologic emergencies are also discussed. Simulation requires a pressurized environment and allows a physician-in-training to be observed directly as he or she evaluates and manages acute neurologic disease. The section concludes with an in-depth guide to developing these teaching scenarios. Traditionally, each simulation has a learner ($\mathcal{L}$) or participant, and a facilitator, or instructor. In addition, there are so-called confederates ($\mathcal{CONF}$), who are individuals other than the patient ($\mathcal{P}$) scripted into the simulation who may provide information for the learner. Examples include family members and medical personnel (e.g., nurse, physician, or respiratory therapist). Such a cast can create a simulated live situation. The room is usually a replica of an emergency room or intensive care unit. Simulation of complex clinical events with changes in vital signs and organ failure usually requires a high-fidelity mannequin or actors. Mannequins provide an array of physiologic responses, including changes in breathing, blood pressure, and pulse, and also pupillary responses and "convulsions." Simulated patients and confederates may be portrayed by medical personnel and actors, and their presence provides a much-needed realism.

Part II is the core of the book. Fifteen acute neurologic emergencies, including complex neuroethical quandaries, are presented in detail, step by step, decision by decision, error after error. Each chapter in this section starts with an explanation of the essence of the discussed neuroemergency (*The Problem Before Us*), followed by a description of the scenario itself (*The Presenting Clinical Problem*), how scenarios can be adjusted to different types of learners (*Adapting the Scenario*), and ends with a discussion of topics for feedback, which are generally focused around errors and pitfalls (*Debriefing*). Scenarios are intended to demonstrate what really goes on in the simulation center and provide a "fly on the wall" experience to the readers. To show the flow of scenarios, we created two additional main headings (*The Ideal Learner* and *The Not-So Ideal Learner*).

The book provides a good number of directives but tries to avoid a "cookbook, bullet-point, algorithmic, or cliff-notes" approach, and each scenario will have to be developed by a team of simulationists. Some things may work in some environments but not others, and nothing in simulation should be etched in stone. Learners' feedback often changes a scenario considerably, and learners may differ. This book, however, intends to give a solid framework to move ahead with this new exciting teaching opportunity.

We realize teaching also requires organizational talent and a good number of technical fixes. We thank the tremendously motivated staff of our simulation center who have allowed us to develop these scenarios. We thank Lea Dacy for her unfailing administrative support but, more importantly, her sharp editorial eye. We thank Jim Rownd for designing the cover showing a learner opposite a patient. Looking at the patient (a fixed and dilated pupil) should lead to a number of actions represented in the hexagonal collection. This deconstruction theme returns in the simulation scenarios. We thank Melanie Tucker from Elsevier for helping us move this project forward and for bringing it to fruition.

For several years, we have run most of these scenarios in our simulation center, and learners can complete between 4 and 6 scenarios per afternoon. It requires a significant commitment from a large number of colleagues, actors, and simulation center staff, and we are very grateful for their support and unbridled enthusiasm. We are convinced—after hearing the experiences of others—that the basic methodology of simulation contributes to best care of patients with an acute neurologic emergency by improving the training of clinicians caring for these patients. This text could serve as a useful reference for those who seek to implement or perfect an existing acute neurology simulation program. To all of you we say good luck!

Sara E. Hocker
Eelco F. M. Wijdicks

Contents

CHAPTER 1

Principles of Simulation

An argument can be made that education in medicine is undergoing a transformative moment and simulation is at the center of it. The value of didactic instruction at the bedside, lectures, and case-based discussions remains untouched, but simulation of disease states and procedures in carefully designed simulation centers is thriving. Simulated disease-specific scenarios test the performance of any healthcare worker using real-time changes, some of which can even occur in response to the actions of the trainee. This continuous interaction is a key component of simulation and reflects acute clinical decision-making while thinking through the consequences of a decision. Simulation of a critical medical situation can be summarized in one word—action![1-4] Decisions are rapid-fire, but the experience is short—a well-planned scenario can be completed in less than 30 minutes.

Simulation is highly structured and objectives are clearly set. Part of the scripted plan involves noting commonly observed trepidations or failures and discussing them in an open, non-threatening, and introspective debriefing. Simulation takes place in designated centers with a complex floorplan. Simulation occurs in multipurpose rooms, usually a replica of an emergency room or intensive care unit. Simulation of clinical events usually requires a high-fidelity mannequin or actors. Mannequins provide an array of physiologic responses, predominantly changes in breathing, blood pressure, and pulse. Actors are often former healthcare workers closely familiar with the simulated disease states and are able to provide some of their key features. Their role in playing patient family members has been particularly rewarding.

Many major academic institutions have established centers with experienced, specifically trained and accredited personnel, and there is major interest to venture further into this field.[5] Moreover, the number of simulation centers is increasing and has become part of a curriculum of medical education for physicians and allied health personnel.[6] It has been recognized that traditional teaching cannot replicate or even approach a well-constructed simulation scenario for teaching acute situations. We will anticipate (and have already seen) that apprenticeship will be complemented with competency-based training. It has become clear that "claimed experience" does not always equal competence—your bedside teacher may not do it right after all those years.[5,7]

There is a growing body of literature, and several textbooks and guidance books have presented the principles of medical simulation.[8-10] There are a number of professional organizations devoted to simulation with training courses and annual meetings. This chapter functions as an introduction to the terminology and principles of simulation.

RATIONALE FOR SIMULATION

Simulation involves teaching technical as well as nontechnical skills. A complicated technical procedure is better first encountered in a patient simulator, working through decision trees and learning from errors along the way. In fact, medical simulation was originally utilized to teach procedural and surgical skills that include cardiopulmonary resuscitation, central line placement, intubation, and mechanical ventilation.[11-16] Another major example was the development of instruction in cardiopulmonary resuscitation with a training mannequin called *Resusci Annie* (a.k.a. Rescue Annie). Training sessions followed by a feedback algorithm were able to successfully and objectively improve technique.[17] Over time, simulation in critical care and anesthesia has become more sophisticated and detailed. Bench-top model training in surgery has been shown to facilitate the acquisition of new skills, and most impressive are the virtual reality laparoscopic trainers and robotic simulation platforms. Devices and standards for teaching have appeared with well-defined algorithms leading to a successful outcome and learning experience.

Most scenarios also try to teach new skills that enable the learner to work individually or lead a team. A simulation can build confidence and allow errors but also may reveal a learner's organizational talent. Learners are placed into an unfamiliar role that, depending on their performance, could result in a marked increase or decrease in self-confidence. Simulation courses are aimed exactly at remedying these insufficiencies. There is therefore a good rationale for simulation, and learners do understand they are in a learning situation and not strictly in an evaluation situation. The goal remains to create a high impact, high value, learning experience.

TERMINOLOGY AND PARTICIPANTS

Programs have developed a unique simulation parlance. The commonly used terminology is shown in Table 1.1. Scenario design must consider learning objectives, fidelity, prebriefing, and debriefing. All scenarios start with a number of objectives with the overall purpose to improve competence in a specific skill. Providing specific learning objectives for every scenario is important because the objectives create a framework by which learners can measure their skill level and opportunities for growth. We use the terms "learning objectives" and "competencies" somewhat interchangeably. The key competencies are the most critical steps required to manage the situation being simulated. The learning objectives necessarily include these key competencies but are typically more comprehensive in scope.

The designation "fidelity" refers to the degree of realism experienced by the learner in a simulation environment and is categorized as high-, medium- and low-fidelity. High-fidelity patient simulators are lifelike, computerized mannequins that can be controlled by the instructors. High-fidelity mannequins can be used

to simulate respiratory difficulties and major changes in vital functions. Most institutions use SimMan3G, which is wireless, self-contained, and offers the opportunity for objective data collection.

The person undergoing training is a "learner" (L) (In the book we will designate them with these symbols). Depending on the scenario and the disease represented, the "simulated patient" (P) can be either a high-fidelity mannequin or an actor coached in the role. The teacher or instructor is sometimes also called "facilitator." "Confederates" $(CONF)$ portray healthcare professionals or family members of the patient. Simulated patients and confederates portrayed by medical personnel and actors provide a much-needed realism. Although confederates in some scenarios portray clinicians or other healthcare professionals instructed to guide and challenge choices made by the learner, they can also represent family members with questions or family members providing additional history. Confederates are able to add appropriate emotions including sadness and anxiety. They may offer clues to the diagnosis by providing a history and can serve as the facilitator's liaison to control the flow of the scenario.

The facilitator outlines to the participants the objectives and tasks, time allotment, orientation to equipment, and the general environment ("prebriefing"). Learners may complete a single scenario or a series of scenarios as part of a larger course. In our experience, four to six scenarios can be completed in a morning or afternoon. Following the scenarios, facilitators lead the learners through a feedback session ("debriefing").

Faculty development is best organized through a structured framework to ensure consistency (and, likely, quality). Some educators advocate a tiered development to enable faculty to grow into "expert simulationists."[15,18–20] The Office of Interprofessional Simulation for Innovative Clinic Practice (University of Alabama, Birmingham) has developed a plan for certification at varying levels, although it currently lacks the authority to mandate certain certification levels.[20] Many simulation centers have recruited interested fellows and faculty and have progressed from mere observation to providing didactics on how to develop a scenario and to actual participation in all components of a simulation scenario. Each tier is reached through peer coaching.

TABLE 1.1 Terminology	
Term	**Meaning**
Learner (L)	Person that undergoes training
Facilitator	Coach, instructor, evaluator
Simulated patient (P)	Actor or mannequin simulating patient
Confederate $(CONF)$	Actor simulating healthcare professional or family member
Objective	Intended result of instruction
Fidelity	Degree of realism
Prebriefing	Orientation, expectation, establishing safe learning environment
Debriefing	Reflection and feedback

PRINCIPLES OF SIMULATION

Simulation-based learning can be set apart from traditional learning models (Figs. 1.1 and 1.2). Traditional learning is mostly passive and comprises lectures, reading, audiovisual material, demonstration

Traditional Learning

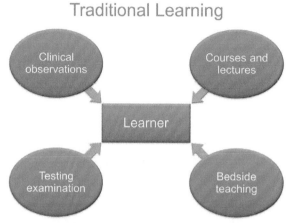

FIG. 1.1 Traditional teaching model.

Simulation-Based Learning

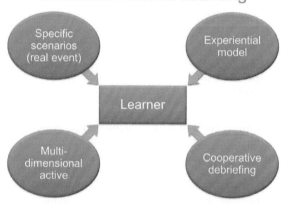

FIG. 1.2 Simulation teaching model.

of the patient, and observation of technical skill. Simulation-based learning is multidimensional and learner-focused. Its characteristic feature is so-called experiential learning. This model offers an experience followed by guided reflection, restatement of what was learned and what could be done differently, which then might result in a changed behavior. The simulation is done with high-simulator fidelity (sophisticated, computerized mannequins mimicking real life), medium-simulator fidelity, or low-simulator fidelity (incorporates a static tool). During these scenarios, the role of facilitator is to coach, instruct, and eventually, provide a level of assessment, where the learner and instructor will discuss together whether the training has achieved its goals. These assessments might involve checklists and scoring systems but also a clinical outcome. Simulation of acute neurology in the emergency department or intensive care unit setting requires multiple steps. These

include problem identification, assessment of targeted learners, goals and objectives, educational strategies, implementation, evaluation, and feedback.[5] Many scenarios have a critical event(s)— pass-or-fail moments that will stop learners in their tracks. Such a prompt aborting of the scenario will then lead to remediation with an often successful result.

Prebriefing

One week before the simulation, trainees receive appropriate prereading materials selected to provide the necessary fund of knowledge to be able to navigate scenarios. This material may include guidelines, editorials, instructional videos, or expert reviews on a topic. Trainees are instructed to carefully review these materials to prepare for the simulation exercise. However, when trainees arrive, they will not know which scenarios they will encounter to avoid too much preparation. Immediately preceding the simulation, trainees meet with the course director who orients them to the simulation center, provides instruction in how to interact with the mannequin and actors (i.e. to avoid the sternal rub or other uncomfortable maneuvers), and introduces the "fiction contract" to learners. The fiction contract is a contract between those executing the simulation and the learner that essentially states:

> We know that this isn't a real patient, but we do our best to make the experience as real as possible. We ask that you do your best to treat it as much like a real patient encounter as possible, which will give you the most learning from the experience.[21]

Learners are also encouraged to 'think aloud', verbalizing their actions and the reasons behind them. All trainees provide informed consent to be videotaped during the prebriefing. The learner and instructor interactions are summarized in Table 1.2.

Scenario Execution and Flow

The simulation technician can alter vital signs remotely at the direction of the facilitator. Teaching staff may wear headsets to facilitate communication during the scenario. Virtually all simulation centers use one-way mirrors, and both the facilitator and confederate wear a headsets through which they communicate. A phone in the room can connect to the instructor, who may portray a consulting physician providing advice, a pharmacist, radiologist, or other medical professional.

Debriefing

Debriefing is the most important component of the simulation exercise because it is here where the learner's experience is reviewed.[22] If the targeted skill was not

TABLE 1.2 Learner-Instructor Interaction	
Learner/Trainee	**Instructor/Facilitator**
• Adheres to 'fiction contract'	• Creative
• Prepared (completed pre-reading, free of external distractions, rested)	• Enthusiastic • Organized • Experienced
• Flexible	• Open to feedback
• Engaged	• Non-judgmental/ compassionate
• Motivated	• Focused on the objectives
• Reflective	• Compassionate

present before the simulated exercise and "the patient is harmed" because of decisions made by the learner, guided reflection is needed. Debriefing allows discussion of step-by-step decision-making in which learners recognize specific pitfalls. This discussion is a major benefit of experiential learning. Immediately following completion of the scenario, the facilitator leads a three-phased, standardized debriefing session that includes (1) the learner's initial reactions to the experience, (2) a detailed discussion of performance, and (3) a summary of key points that may be applied in clinical practice. Learning objectives are reinforced and errors and challenges addressed. If pertinent, learners can observe key moments of their scenario on video playback during the debriefing session.

These complex scenarios demand medical knowledge, leadership (to manage the team during the simulated emergency), and clinical skill. The stress level during the performance is also identified and addressed. Debriefing sessions should avoid excessive criticism or mocking of learners. Discussion should never focus on the poor performance of the learner. An autocratic attitude can seriously upset the learner and, ultimately, destroy a program. Debriefings should preferably stress a few key points and avoid negativism. All in all, competence and performance can be deconstructed in four parts (Fig. 1.3).

VALIDATION

Simulation can provide significant educational benefits. Whether it is substantially more useful than traditional teaching is, however, unconfirmed. Before these

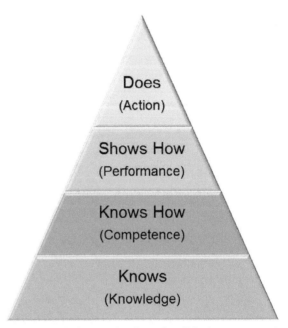

FIG. 1.3 Miller's triangle of clinical assessment. (Adapted from Miller GE. The assessment of clinical skills /competence/performance. Academic Med 1990;65: S63–S67.)

programs become mandated as curriculum, prospective studies should examine whether the experience actually improves skills. Simulation is costly and requires a substantial time commitment from instructors and paid actors. Studies may have the burden of proof to demonstrate effect on physician performance and, eventually and far more ambitiously, on patient outcome.[23,24] Most assessments of simulation can be done by measuring content validity and construct validity. Content validity usually refers to whether the test is representative of what needs to be assessed. Construct validity indicates whether the test actually measures what it has to measure. The measurement of educational tools remains notoriously difficult, and this applies in particular to simulation.[24] Multiple self-assessment scales as well as skills have been developed and validated. Checklists (and a requirement to meet or exceed a minimum passing score) may be developed for each simulation scenario. These checklists may vary in number of items checked but ideally should consist of 10 or fewer to enhance focus and avoid complexity. Immediate fail may be used in situations of gross negligence (e.g., diagnosing brain death in a markedly hypothermic patient). Data can be analyzed using interrater reliability making use of the mean kappa coefficient. With testing of different specialties, linear-regression models can assess relationships between specialties. However, even if differences are significant, certain failures or lapses may not be consequential, again requiring careful vetting and review before items for assessment are introduced in checklists.

Teamwork skills become important when there are multiple participants in the simulated setting.[14,25] Some studies have used a combination of self-assessment and external ratings by experts. Nonetheless, the quality of evidence on simulation-based neurology education is generally nonexistent, or the level of reporting is poor. Rating scales can assess a number of important findings, and these scales should be generalizable to be applicable to all scenarios. Items that can be rated are (1) adequate communication and verbalization of activities, (2) adapting a plan when a situation changes, (3) requesting external assistance when appropriate, (4) resolution of conflicts that can impair team performance, (5) responding to potential errors or complications with procedures, (6) avoidance of fixation on isolated abnormalities, (7) inclusion of other aspects of care, (8) appropriate triage, (9) ability to maintain focus on the critical situation, and (10) adequate verbal communication to bystanders and family members and clear explanation of the critical situation.

These validity scales have been useful, but learners have voiced concerns and barriers. Many doubt their preparedness or ability to deal with certain situations and fear an embarrassing performance. Goldberg et al. have established "Las Vegas rules" for their simulation center, i.e., "whatever happens in the simulation lab stays in the simulation lab." Periods belong *inside* quotation marks.[26] They emphasize that no one should judge or report the performance of a learner, and learners are forewarned that difficult, undesirable events might be part of a planned scenario. Their goal is to make the learner understand that while things often go well in clinical practice, the simulation center exists to educate learners to manage situations in which adverse, unexpected events occur.[26] This approach has greatly improved learner satisfaction.

THE LIMITS, CHALLENGES, AND CONTROVERSIES OF SIMULATION

The most important challenge is to achieve "buy-in" from departments. Simulation programs cannot proceed without significant motivation. It requires recognition of key players and support to learners for attendance at these educational programs.[25]

Another important challenge is to match the fidelity to task. Simulation does not have to recreate a perfect clinical environment to be useful. Some situations can be best simulated with actors portraying patients and confederates. Simulation skeptics often argue that the exercises are inauthentic, not unique, not proven better, too costly, and likely to teach overaggressiveness. Their argument is significant doubt that "actors" can convincingly portray disease and much of it may seem contrived. However, precision in portrayal is not necessary and learners are not really bothered by it. It is far more important to create a realistic environment and a specific situation for the learner to navigate. The creation of a realistic environment requires time and, often, dry runs to identify flaws in the methodology.

There are other potential barriers. Some residents and fellows object to this type of teaching, particularly when it is scheduled at the end of residency because they see it as exposing their weaknesses. Simulation center instructors have also recognized that hypercriticism of the student may lead to complex emotions and negative attitudes toward learning. Simulation scenarios can create impulsiveness, inflexibility, and even later conflict within learners if the situation gets out of control.

Emergencies are often best characterized as low-frequency, high-demand, and resource-intense events. The physician may have difficulty recalling best practices for a given scenario. In real life, they may be asked to handle clinical situations typically handled by certain specialists, resulting in additional fear of incompetence. Given the dire consequences of missteps in medicine, it is a given that any and all teaching methods in medical education will induce some degree of stress in the learners. Whether the stress level is acceptable depends in part on how well it helps learners to improve their competency. In this sense, the stress induced in a simulation exercise is preferable to the stress induced in the Socratic method, which relies on probing and leading to make connections between certain pieces of information. Most certainly, it is infinitely preferable to "pimping," a perversion of the Socratic method described in a tongue-in-cheek JAMA essay by Brancati in 1989.[27] This undesirable method is a form of directed learning where the teacher asks questions— often arcane or obscure questions designed to confuse and silence the learners—in quick succession. Promoted as a way to cultivate humility, it actually humiliates and harasses learners to create an extraordinarily stressful learning environment. No learner should be overwhelmed with a flurry of medical and neurologic instabilities or a patient who is rapidly declining or spiraling toward a fatal outcome. All physicians experience a high level of stress fueled by fear of failure, fear of an uninformative exam, and fear of a lapse in diagnostics and care with these unanticipated emergencies and there is a possibility of decline in confidence and increase in frustration. Physicians who go through the experience of a real high-pressure medical emergency may expose their own deficiencies.

One approach to simulation is to make simulation competitive between teams. The SimWars competition has been held during professional meetings with an audience voting for the team with the best performance making use of judges. A current curriculum involves emergency medicine cases alone and is mostly focused on stabilization and who to consult. Some cases are overdramatized with excited, screaming patients, agitated anxious family members, arrogant consultants, and a number of other built-in distractions. Whether a good dose of entertainment is the way forward is debatable, and we suspect the more serious educators will disagree with this approach.

Likewise, simulation of death has been a source of debate and controversy among simulation educators.[28] Although simulating death can be a powerful learning tool, it should not be used punitively. It can, however, be used if the learner's action leads to a life-threatening complication, for example, after administration of the wrong drug or potentially lethal dose of the right drug. Some educators advocate against allowing the death of the simulated patient in exercises for early learners such as medical students, although simulator death may be effective in more complex scenarios for advanced learners. Other arguments against simulating death include the psychological safety of learners and possible reluctance to participate in future simulation training.[29] It can be argued that careful, prolonged debriefing mitigates these concerns, but most experts agree that creating "no-win" scenarios, regardless of the case, does not enhance any teaching experience.[30,31]

Another controversy in simulation is the use of deception. Some simulation scenarios have confederates make deliberate mistakes or have a team leader make an obvious mistake to elicit a response from the other learners. Such a modification in simulation should be discouraged; it tends to create a "reality show" rather than a serious teaching environment.[32] Simulation is also not an ideal environment for teaching learners how to push back against authority. Some have rightfully argued that deception is more problematic when learners are not informed in advance that one of the learning goals is to examine how they respond to authority.[32,33]

Simulation requires substantial resources including time, space, money, staff, expertise, and a plan to ensure sustainability. Nevertheless, many major academic institutions have centers in place with experienced personnel, and there is major interest to venture into this field. The ultimate challenge is to demonstrate that simulation-based research translates to training in real patient-care settings. Recent studies have confirmed improved in-house cardiac resuscitation after simulation.[34–36] However, there have also been some disturbing revelations. Simulation has shown that decision-making failures can be attributed to disregard of the severity of the crisis, knowledge deficit, lack of reasoning capability, or inability to communicate, prioritizing fixation on one single symptom to the exclusion of more important ones, and, most hazardous, behavioral attitudes such as impulsiveness, inflexibility, egotism, or what has been called an "unguided missile." Nonetheless, all these challenges can be easily overcome when the stakeholders remain positive, friendly, and create a durable experience. Simulation is here to stay if the culture is cooperative and supportive.

CONCLUSIONS

Simulation requires substantial resources including time, space, money, staff, and expertise.[33] The role of the instructors is important, and reinforcement and facilitation, including verbal praise during debriefing, are necessary. The debriefing session should emphasize key competencies and highlight good decisions, as well as judgment errors. A lack of positive feedback can cause the learner to fail dramatically and will rapidly lead to demotivation and loss of the program's effectiveness. Effective instruction in neurosimulation requires a new sort of creative teacher with energy, commitment, and compassion.

Operation techniques are now very commonly taught through simulation before residents and fellows are allowed a real-life experience. Medical clinical decision making is in development and has been identified as a teaching opportunity.[33] In essence, no one simply wants to be told how to do it and follow some instruction—it is preferable to have the full (the good and the bad) experience and simulation provides a safe space in which to provide it. Simulation in medicine has steadily grown and gained acceptance as an educational tool. Now, simulation in neurology is the logical next step.[33]

REFERENCES

1. Issenberg SB. The scope of simulation-based healthcare education. *Simul Healthc.* 2006;1:203–208.

2. Issenberg SB, McGaghie WC, Hart IR, et al. Simulation technology for health care professional skills training and assessment. *JAMA.* 1999;282:861–866.

3. McGaghie WC, Issenberg SB, Petrusa ER, et al. A critical review of simulation-based medical education research: 2003–2009. *Med Educ.* 2010;44:50–63.

4. Ryall T, Judd BK, Gordon CJ. Simulation-based assessments in health professional education: a systematic review. *J Multidiscip Healthc.* 2016;9:69–82.

5. Gaba DM, Howard SK, Fish KJ, et al. Simulation-based training in anesthesia crisis resource management (ACRM): a decade of experience. *Simul Gaming.* 2001;32:175–193.

6. Levine AI, DeMaria JS, Schwartz AD, et al. *The Comprehensive Textbook of Healthcare Simulation.* New York: Springer; 2013.

7. Spadaro S, Karbing DS, Fogagnolo A, et al. Simulation training for residents focused on mechanical ventilation: a randomized trial using mannequin-based versus computer-based simulation. *Simul Healthc.* 2017;12:349–355.

8. Dunn WF, ed. *Simulators in Critical Care and Beyond.* 2nd ed. Mount Prospect, IL: Society of Critical Care Medicine; 2009.

9. Jacobson L, Okuda Y, Godwin SA, eds. *SimWars Simulation Case Book: Emergency Medicine.* 1st ed. Cambridge, U.K: Cambridge University Press; 2015. Cambridge Medicine.

10. Wilson L, Wittmann-Price R, eds. *Review Manual for the Certified Healthcare Simulation Educator Exam.* 1st ed. New York: Springer; 2014:442.

11. Ali S, Qandeel M, Ramakrishna R, et al. Virtual simulation in enhancing procedural training for fluoroscopy-guided lumbar puncture: a pilot study. *Acad Radiol.* 2018;25: 235–239.

12. Barsuk JH, McGaghie WC, Cohen ER, et al. Simulation-based mastery learning reduces complications during central venous catheter insertion in a medical intensive care unit. *Crit Care Med.* 2009;37:2697–2701.

13. Edelson DP, Litzinger B, Arora V, et al. Improving in-hospital cardiac arrest process and outcomes with performance debriefing. *Arch Intern Med.* 2008;168:1063–1069.

14. Malec JF, Torsher LC, Dunn WF, et al. The mayo high performance teamwork scale: reliability and validity for evaluating key crew resource management skills. *Simul Healthc.* 2007;2:4–10.

15. Nestel D. Ten years of simulation in healthcare: a thematic analysis of editorials. *Simul Healthc.* 2017;12:326–331.

16. Wayne DB, Didwania A, Feinglass J, et al. Simulation-based education improves quality of care during cardiac arrest team responses at an academic teaching hospital: a case-control study. *Chest.* 2008;133:56–61.

17. Preusch MR, Bea F, Roggenbach J, et al. Resuscitation Guidelines 2005: does experienced nursing staff need training and how effective is it? *Am J Emerg Med.* 2010; 28:477–484.

18. Leslie K, Baker L, Egan-Lee E, et al. Advancing faculty development in medical education: a systematic review. *Acad Med.* 2013;88:1038–1045.

19. Nehring WM, Wexler T, Hughes F, et al. Faculty development for the use of high-fidelity patient simulation: a systematic review. *Int J Health Sci Edu.* 2013;1:34.

20. Peterson DT, Watts PI, Epps CA, et al. Simulation faculty development: a tiered approach. *Simul Healthc.* 2017;12: 254–259.

21. Rudolph JW, Raemer DB, Simon R. Establishing a safe container for learning in simulation: the role of the presimulation briefing. *Simul Healthc.* 2014;9:339–349.

22. Zigmont JJ, Kappus LJ, Sudikoff SN. The 3D model of debriefing: defusing, discovering, and deepening. *Semin Perinatol.* 2011;35:52–58.

23. Salas D, Wilson KA, Lazzara EH, et al. Simulation-based training for patient safety: 10 principles that matter. *J Patient Saf.* 2008;4:3–8.

24. Weller J, Shulruf B, Torrie J, et al. Validation of a measurement tool for self-assessment of teamwork in intensive care. *Br J Anaesth.* 2013;111:460–467.

25. Piquette D, LeBlanc VR. Five questions critical care educators should ask about simulation-based medical education. *Clin Chest Med.* 2015;36:469–479.

26. Goldberg AT, Katz D, Levine AI, et al. The importance of deception in simulation: an imperative to train in realism. *Simul Healthc.* 2015;10:386–387.

27. Brancati FL. The art of pimping. *JAMA.* 1989;262:89–90.

28. Corvetto MA, Taekman JM. To die or not to die? A review of simulated death. *Simul Healthc.* 2013;8:8–12.

29. Fraser K, Huffman J, Ma I, et al. The emotional and cognitive impact of unexpected simulated patient death: a randomized controlled trial. *Chest.* 2014;145:958–963.

30. Calhoun AW, Gaba DM. Live or let die: new developments in the ongoing debate over mannequin death. *Simul Healthc.* 2017;12:279–281.

31. Goldberg A, Samuelson S, Khelemsky Y, et al. Exposure to simulated mortality affects resident performance during assessment scenarios. *Simul Healthc.* 2017;12:282–288.

32. Truog RD, Meyer EC. Deception and death in medical simulation. *Simul Healthc.* 2013;8:1–3.

33. Dieckmann P, Lippert A, Glavin R, et al. When things do not go as expected: scenario life savers. *Simul Healthc.* 2010;5:219–225.

34. Gruber C, Nabecker S, Wohlfarth P, et al. Evaluation of airway management associated hands-off time during cardiopulmonary resuscitation: a randomized manikin follow-up study. *Scand J Trauma Resusc Emerg Med.* 2013; 21:10.

35. Taelman DG, Huybrechts SA, Peersman W, et al. Quality of resuscitation by first responders using the 'public access resuscitator': a randomized manikin study. *Eur J Emerg Med.* 2014;21:409–417.

36. Wutzler A, Bannehr M, von Ulmenstein S, et al. Performance of chest compressions with the use of a new audio-visual feedback device: a randomized manikin study in health care professionals. *Resuscitation.* 2015;87: 81–85.

CHAPTER 2

Simulation of Acute Neurology

Neurology has many subspecialties. Among these, acute neurology (or neurocritical care) stands out because it involves acute care of disorders that are potentially life threatening or that may lead to major permanent disability. In addition, multisystem care is anticipated in acute neurologic conditions and is often disease specific. The care of the multitude of these problems requires close cooperation with emergency medicine physicians, neurosurgeons, and infectious disease consultants but also rehabilitation physicians and palliative care specialists. These numerous links to other specialties open up a wide range of simulation possibilities.[1–6]

It is no exaggeration to say that current curricula do not guarantee adequate exposure to major neurologic emergencies for physicians in training simply because these emergencies occur infrequently and at all hours of the day.[7,8] The key question is whether simulation can fill this void. Simulation of acute neurology, compared with other emergency specialties, is in its infancy.[9] Simulation challenges the traditional didactic methods of classroom lectures and direct observation of trainees' clinical skills. However, comparing these two educational methods for efficacy would be cumbersome in the absence of established metrics. Moreover, not all acute neurologic illnesses are conducive to simulation simply because specific technology is not available or actors are not able to reasonably mimic the disorder.

In this chapter, we introduce the rationale for simulation of acute neurology including future opportunities. Simulation of acute neurology and neurocritical care is achievable. Acute neurology can be simulated as long as scenarios concentrate on management of the disorder rather than portrayal of neurologic signs. Simulation of acute neurologic conditions is far from being established and standard. Adjustments to scenarios—mostly major improvements rather than simple tweaks—are expected in institutions working through a simulation program and each institution will have a number of specific challenges and preferences.

TEACHING ACUTE NEUROLOGY

Simulation in acute neurology must center on clinical decision-making.[9] These decisions may involve developing a plan of action, administering appropriate drugs, interpreting neuroimaging, making a clinical diagnosis, and understanding and addressing systemic complications related to acute neurologic injury. Scenarios can be built to foster a sense of urgency, while teaching avoidance of errors[11,12] and actions to address the intricacies of cerebral resuscitation. Morbidity and mortality meetings offer good ideas for building scenarios (Chapter 3), but simulation must go beyond teaching near misses or errors to focus on recognition of difficult presentations and how to work rapidly through a differential diagnosis.[13] Teachable scenarios may include recognition of imminent neuromuscular respiratory failure, recognition of a deteriorating patient with an acute brain lesion, and treatment of refractory status epilepticus. One area in which simulation might outshine all other teaching methods is the area of interpersonal communications (i.e., communication with patients, family members, and other medical staff). For example, scenarios can point out the unique challenges involved in managing a patient emergency while fielding questions from their family, giving "bad news," or discussing brain death. This type of role-play can reinforce important communication techniques and strategies.

When it comes to teaching acute neurology, there are both opportunities and roadblocks. First, its urgency may not be appreciated (enough) by physicians. Second, opportunities to teach decision-making skills at the point of care, and management of critical neurologic states rarely occur in clinical practice, and third, what defines "competency" in handling these acute situations is unknown. Most problematically, major components of the neurologic examination do not lend themselves to any form of simulation, and as mentioned in the previous chapter, the costs and labor involved are high. Finally, neuroemergencies have been duly established as an entrustable professional activity (EPA) correlated to milestones within the Accreditation Council for

Graduate Medical Education core competencies. Unlike the other five EPAs, however, neuroemergency EPAs are not consistently taught.[5,7,8,10]

Acute neurology as a specialty encompasses diseases with high levels of morbidity and mortality. The morbidity of neurologic illness involves the personalities and emotional lives of our patients. Discussing goals of care and ethical conflicts with acutely distraught patients and families in the setting of acute neurologic illness—where some time pressure may exist—requires practice but can be taught. Video playback documents the learner's body language, use of medical jargon, and handling of ethical dilemmas. Such complex personal interplays, not infrequently seen in emergency settings, can only be created in a simulation center and not in general teaching rooms.

APPLICATION OF SIMULATION TO ACUTE NEUROLOGY

Simulation-based education in general practice correlates positively with physician performance and even patient outcomes.[15,16] Incorporating neurology-specific scenarios into simulation can ensure that specific EPAs are met. Simulation provides an artificial environment in which to manage neurologic emergencies, choose appropriate tests, and also to hone skills and strategies for communicating with family members. Effective learning often occurs when physicians err while facing neurologic emergencies. In contrast to traditional teaching methods, simulation can induce a stress response that very effectively mimics what learners will eventually feel when faced with a "real" emergency, an unknown clinical situation in flux, or a complication as a result of treatment decisions or an error. However, simulation is not all about "doing" (i.e., performing a physical examination); it often involves focused "thinking" (e.g., interpretation of the clinical history, neurophysiology, and neuroimaging).

Under the direction of a creative, committed instructor, neurosimulation can assume as much urgency as any other critical care simulation (e.g., cardiac arrhythmia, cardiopulmonary resuscitation, polytrauma). Neurosimulation presents the principles of brain protection and exposes learners to largely unfamiliar drugs and side effects (e.g., osmotic diuretics, antiseizure drugs, and thrombolytics). It can also provide a window into end-of-life care for a comatose patient, which differs significantly from general palliative care measures.

Setup and Equipment

Simulation of acute neurology requires rooms and hardware currently standard in most simulation centers. The setup and rooms needed are shown in Fig. 2.1. Successful learners will be busy from start to finish of the exercise. Instructors will use the Sim man when appropriate and specifically when pulmonary complications are part of the scenario (Fig. 2.2). Some scenarios such as trauma (Chapter 4) lend themselves best to demonstration of team work and leadership (Fig. 2.3).

How to Portray Neurologic Disease?

Elusive, mysterious, and only for well-trained neurologists, the neurologic examination has been considered the "crown jewel" of physical examination. How then is it even possible to simulate such a complex examination? Would any attempt at imitating a finding be ridiculous (or awkward at best)? Would acting it out devalue the beauty of the examination? Is it not already laughable or painful to watch actors portray a patient with a neurologic disease (with the possible exceptions of Daniel Day Lewis in *My Left Foot* and Emmanuelle Riva in *Amour*)? Would cynics say that only psychogenic weakness can be imitated?[17,18]

These valid criticisms cannot be fully countered, but the current experience is quite different—indeed better—than what most of us initially expected. Simulation centers with mannequins, actors, and well-prepared instructors can create a very teachable situation.

Actors (often experienced nurses) can do more than most physicians intuitively believe, and we and others have been impressed with what they are able to simulate (Fig. 2.4).[19,20] As long as scenarios focus on a few major signs, several classic neuroemergencies can be imitated. Examples of applications to simulation in acute neurology are shown in Table 2.1. Several disorders can be taught quite nicely, and while the teaching of specific scenarios is further discussed in the second part of this book, we offer the following examples.

To encourage learners to recognize and manage the early complications of aneurysmal subarachnoid hemorrhage, an actor describes symptoms when asked (Chapter 7). When the learner elicits a history of thunderclap headache and orders a CT scan, the scan shows diffuse subarachnoid blood and early hydrocephalus. The monitor displays severe hypertension with a BP of 190/140 mmHg. Shortly after antihypertensive drug administration, the patient suddenly develops a severe headache, has a "seizure," and becomes unresponsive with a Cushing reflex. At this point, the learner ideally

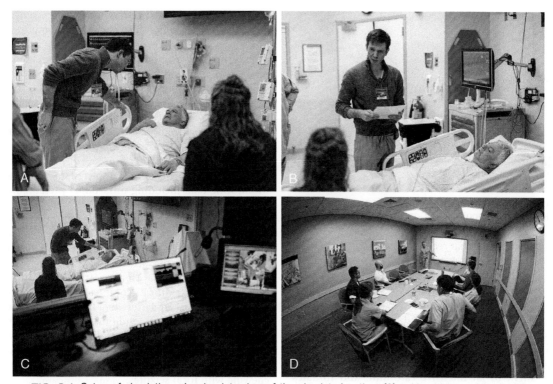

FIG. 2.1 Setup of simulation, showing interview of the simulated patient **(A)**, taking history of family **(B)** Control room **(C)**. Debriefing room allowing discussion of the scenario and also reviewing of taped interactions **(D)**.

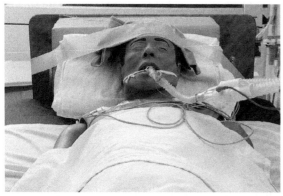

FIG. 2.2 Example of a simulation mannequin (SimMan 3G, Laerdal Medical, Wappingers Falls, NY).

recognizes aneurysmal rebleeding, reexamines the patient, and assesses the airway. Concerned about progressive hydrocephalus, the learner should request a CT scan and neurosurgical evaluation. At this point, if the learner states that emergent cerebrospinal fluid (CSF) diversion is needed, the scenario ends. Alternatively, if

the resident does not answer appropriately, the heart rate drops to 30 bpm and BP increases to 230/110 mmHg resulting in respiratory and circulatory arrest. This scenario highlights two serious early complications of subarachnoid hemorrhage: rebleeding and hydrocephalus. Teaching points include early avoidance of beta blockade, as the patient is at risk for bradycardia due to a Cushing reflex during rebleeding; worsening hydrocephalus; early aggressive blood pressure control to reduce the risk of rebleeding; and recognition of hydrocephalus and the need for emergent CSF diversion.

We found myasthenic crisis to be ideally suited to simulating neuromuscular respiratory weakness (Chapter 11). Neuromuscular respiratory failure can be simulated by an actor instructed to use interrupted speech while catching a breath, to lean forward, to elevate the shoulders, and to breathe paradoxically in the supine position. Moisture is applied to the actor's forehead while tachycardia and hypertension are displayed on the monitor. If this is not recognized as imminent failure and appropriately managed, the patient develops frank

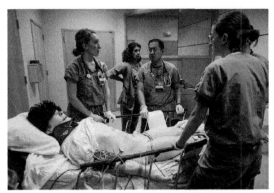

FIG. 2.3 Setup of trauma mannequin emphasizing team work, individual responsibilities, and leadership skills.

respiratory failure that requires intubation. While the learner communicates and writes admission orders, the patient becomes drowsier, the heart rate increases, and oxygen saturation declines. Where noninvasive ventilation may have previously sufficed, the learner now must call for emergent intubation and deal with the risks therein including apnea and cardiovascular collapse. If the learner recognizes impending neuromuscular respiratory failure, triages the patient to an intensive care unit, and initiates noninvasive ventilation or endotracheal intubation and mechanical ventilation, the patient survives without complications.

Treatment for status epilepticus can be taught in different ways (Chapter 12). The patient may develop refractory shock after receiving lorazepam, fosphenytoin, and pentobarbital loading for refractory status epilepticus. Laboratory evaluation can show a marked metabolic acidosis with an elevated serum lactate level, hyperosmolality, and increased osmolar gap. The teaching point for the learner is to appreciate that propylene-glycol toxicity can complicate a barbiturate coma and, consequently, to substitute another drug for the pento-barbital infusion. Alternatively, the patient may develop a cardiac arrhythmia during fosphenytoin loading, which, if recognized, should prompt the learner to discontinue the infusion and treat with an appropriate alternative.

Focal status epilepticus in the setting of epidural empyema can also be simulated. The actor is instructed to keep his eyes open and stare forward, repetitively move the fingers or arm on one side of the body while not moving the other, and remain unresponsive. Ultimately, the actor may be prompted to have generalized stiffening; clenching of the teeth; extension of the neck, trunk, and legs; and flexion

of the previously motionless side. Fever may be shown. Teaching points can include the importance of CT scan before lumbar puncture, empiric initiation of antimicrobial agents, and indications for emergent electroencephalography. An ideal neurosimulator would show a number of eye-movement abnormalities (nystagmus, ocular bobbing) and changes in eye position with vestibular stimulation. Different coordinated, synchronized motor movements (decorticate, decerebrate posturing) could potentially be simulated with a computer monitor displaying preset EEG patterns, transcranial Doppler data, and other monitoring data including intracranial pressure from a placed probe.

Portraying aphasia and hemiparesis through neurosimulation is perhaps inadvisable, but global aphasia (not Wernicke's aphasia) can be successfully directed simply by having the actor say one repeated word such as "no," or "good." Hemiparesis and hemiplegia can be shown as a drift or complete flaccidity, respectively (testing of muscles for hemiparesis would show give-way weakness, and thus, we avoid this level of detail). Motor movements are limited, but convulsions with eye deviation could convey sufficient reality. The same applies to picking behaviors and chewing with focal seizures.

However, certain findings cannot be imitated; these are clonus, pyramidal weakness, increased tone, many movement disorders, and gait ataxia. Any of these would be indistinguishable from functional disorders. Traumatic brain injury can be extended to polytrauma but also may teach initial management of intracranial hypertension, prevention of further spinal cord injury, and initial resuscitation measures (e.g., which fluids to use, appropriate blood pressure targets, and best practices for monitoring potential instability of vital signs). A team approach may be best for practicing a level 1 trauma.

How to Teach Successful Family Conferences on Patients With Neurologic Injury?

Simulation centers are ideal for role-play with carefully constructed scenarios (Chapter 18). Such role-play can include leading a family conference for a patient with a catastrophic neurologic disorder. Families play large roles in decision-making, and conflicts can be easily simulated. The importance of these interactions cannot be emphasized enough because (1) they are unique, (2) they require clear explanations of the neurologic disability in lay terms, and (3) they draw on the real-life experiences of

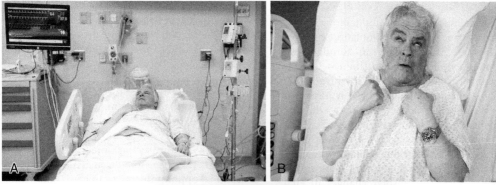

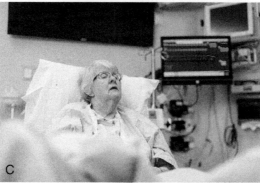

FIG. 2.4 Examples of portrayals by actors (**A**, stroke with hemiplegia and neglect favoring one side; **B**, seizure with flexed arms and rolled-up eyes; **C**, myasthenia with ptosis, bifacial palsy, and shortness of breath).

neurointensivists or emergency physicians who do this every day. One scenario might be a conference with the family of a comatose patient with a catastrophic hemorrhage. Confederates can portray estranged siblings fighting about the plan of treatment based on their own values. The learner must (1) explain the families' role as surrogate decision maker to them while emphasizing that the focus should be on what the patient would want, (2) help family members identify what their loved one would find acceptable if she could speak for herself, (3) allow family members to speak individually about their concerns, and (4) identify a course of action acceptable to all. This scenario can play out in many different ways. If the learner sides with one faction or the other, reinforcing the divide between them and angering the other party, he or she must then defuse the situation created. Others may lose control of the discussion, get lost in the individual beliefs of both surrogates, and ultimately, fail to redirect the focus to the wishes of the patient. The addition of time urgency to the discussion can significantly alter the difficulty level of these scenarios.

TABLE 2.1
Neurologic Signs Suitable for Portrayal by Actors
• Forced gaze deviation and apraxia of eyelid opening
• Facial twitching (cheek)
• Hemianopia
• Vertical eye movements only (locked-in syndrome)
• Neck stiffness
• Global aphasia (mute or only "no" or "good")
• Complete paralysis—arm[a]
• Complete paralysis—leg[a]
• Complete paraparesis[a]
• Sensory level (to be detected with pinprick)[a]
• Neglect and anosognosia
• Seizures (some types)
• Myoclonic twitches, asterixis (possibly)
• Accessory respiratory muscle activation and paradoxical breathing (neuromuscular respiratory failure)
• Posturing

[a] Pain stimuli are mentioned—not applied.

What Props and Devices Are Available?

Mannequins are commonly used for training,[19,21,22] although they are not suited for simulation of most neurologic diseases. Mannequins can simulate eye opening, blinking, pupillary changes (limited to reactivity and symmetry), and "shaking" or shivering. If necessary, mannequins can "talk" when an instructor in the control center serves as the "voice-over," offering simple comments such as "it hurt so bad, never had this before." In some situations, such as subarachnoid hemorrhage, they can make the mannequin moan as if from a headache. Independent of the mannequin, the simulation software can display changes in vital signs, which can include cardiac arrhythmias (e.g., during phenytoin loading), hypotension (e.g., sepsis with bacterial meningitis), hypothermia (e.g., myxedema coma), and hypoxemia (e.g., after seizure).

In acute neurology, neuroimaging (mostly CT and CT angiogram, chest and cervical X-rays) should be available on a workstation in the room. Laboratory values are presented on paper or recorded on a whiteboard as requested by the learner. Pupillary abnormalities can be displayed on a photograph but frequently do not add enough diagnostic value to justify the reduction in realism.

Moulage is useful to show skin abnormalities. Some examples, including needle tracks in a comatose patient, make-up rash in encephalitis or bacterial meningitis, and pre-made sweat formulas, are available to portray patients with acute neuromuscular respiratory failure, and edible moulage can mimic a tongue bite from a seizure. The use of props requires innovative thinking and a willingness to suspend reality, but learners accept these limitations.

Future Challenges in Neurosimulation

The question remains if we can build (or need) a neurosimulator. An ideal neurosimulator would be able to demonstrate eye-movement abnormalities (e.g., nystagmus, ocular bobbing) and changes in eye position with vestibular stimulation. It should be able to simulate coordinated, synchronized motor movements (decorticate or decerebrate posturing). The computerized neurosimulator could theoretically show preset EEG patterns, transcranial Doppler data, and intracranial pressure from a placed probe. Both lumbar puncture and ophthalmoscope models are already commercially available, but whether a neurosimulator (or any specialist-driven simulator) is financially feasible is unknown.[23–26] It remains to be seen whether neurologic findings are conducive to computer simulation.

Other opportunities have presented themselves, and there is interest in using telemedicine for simulation. Simulation of acute ischemic stroke using telestroke has been validated as an instrument to improve skills.[27]

CONCLUSIONS

As outlined in Chapter 1, simulation, even as currently practiced, requires substantial resources, including time, space, money, staff, and expertise, to maintain sustainability.[28] Instructors must be creative and committed. However, for the first time in neurology, educational opportunities exist to teach neuroemergencies safely. The challenge remains to write a scenario that is useful to the learner—not just a bag of tricks seeking to entrap him or her. In our experience, the response of the learners has been positive. Indeed, many commented that they entered into the exercise so fully that they forgot it was a simulation. One learner said, "Simulation makes me nervous—it is unreal." Actors can provide the basic neurologic findings needed to make a scenario successful. While learners know it is not a real stroke or seizure, they clearly and immediately recognize it as such and proceed with treatment. This book will show how these scenarios may effectively simulate situations encountered in acute neurology and how they have worked for us.

REFERENCES

1. Dhar R, Rajajee V, Finley Caulfield A, et al. The state of neurocritical care fellowship training and attitudes toward accreditation and certification: a survey of neurocritical care fellowship program directors. *Front Neurol.* 2017;8: 548.
2. James ML, Dority J, Gray MC, et al. Survey of anesthesiologists practicing in American neurointensive care units as neurointensivists. *J Neurosurg Anesthesiol.* 2014;26:11–16.
3. Marcolini EG, Seder DB, Bonomo JB, et al. The present state of neurointensivist training in the United States: a comparison to other critical care training programs. *Crit Care Med.* 2018;46:307–315.
4. Markandaya M, Thomas KP, Jahromi B, et al. The role of neurocritical care: a brief report on the survey results of neurosciences and critical care specialists. *Neurocrit Care.* 2012;16:72–81.
5. Napolitano LM, Rajajee V, Gunnerson KJ, et al. Physician training in critical care in the United States: update 2018. *J Trauma Acute Care Surg.* 2018;84:963–971.
6. Wijdicks EF. The history of neurocritical care. *Handb Clin Neurol.* 2017;140:3–14.
7. Lerner DP, Kim J, Izzy S. Neurocritical care education during residency: opinions (NEURON) study. *Neurocrit Care.* 2017;26:115–118.

8. Moore FG, Chalk C. How well does neurology residency mirror practice? *Can J Neurol Sci.* 2005;32:472−476.

9. Papangelou A, Ziai W. The birth of neuro-simulation. *Neurocrit Care.* 2010;13:167−168.

10. Sheth KN, Drogan O, Manno E, et al. Neurocritical care education during neurology residency: AAN survey of US program directors. *Neurology.* 2012;78:1793−1796.

11. Dworetzky BA, Peyre S, Bubrick EJ, et al. Interprofessional simulation to improve safety in the epilepsy monitoring unit. *Epilepsy Behav.* 2015;45:229−233.

12. Salas D, Wilson KA, Lazzara EH, et al. Simulation-based training for patient safety: 10 principles that matter. *J Patient Saf.* 2008;4:3−8.

13. Stone J. Morbidity and mortality meetings for neurologists. *Pract Neurol.* 2008;8:278−279.

14. Kelly MA, Hager P, Gallagher R. What matters most? Students' rankings of simulation components that contribute to clinical judgment. *J Nurs Educ.* 2014;53:97−101.

15. Brydges R, Hatala R, Zendejas B, et al. Linking simulation-based educational assessments and patient-related outcomes: a systematic review and meta-analysis. *Acad Med.* 2015;90:246−256.

16. Cook DA. How much evidence does it take? A cumulative meta-analysis of outcomes of simulation-based education. *Med Educ.* 2014;48:750−760.

17. Hocker S, Schumacher D, Mandrekar J, Wijdicks EFM. Testing confounders in brain death determination: a new simulation model. *Neurocrit Care.* 2015;23:401−408.

18. MacDougall BJ, Robinson JD, Kappus L, et al. Simulation-based training in brain death determination. *Neurocrit Care.* 2014;21:383−391.

19. Micieli G, Cavallini A, Santalucia P, et al. Simulation in neurology. *Neurol Sci.* 2015;36:1967−1971.

20. Musacchio Jr MJ, Smith AP, McNeal CA, et al. Neurocritical care skills training using a human patient simulator. *Neurocrit Care.* 2010;13:169−175.

21. Braksick SA, Kashani K, Hocker S. Neurology education for critical care fellows using high-fidelity simulation. *Neurocrit Care.* 2017;26:96−102.

22. Ermak DM, Bower DW, Wood J, et al. Incorporating simulation technology into a neurology clerkship. *J Am Osteopath Assoc.* 2013;113:628−635.

23. Barsuk JH, Cohen ER, Vozenilek JA, et al. Simulation-based education with mastery learning improves paracentesis skills. *J Grad Med Educ.* 2012;4:23−27.

24. Gupta DK, Khandker N, Stacy K, et al. Utility of combining a simulation-based method with a lecture-based method for fundoscopy training in neurology residency. *JAMA Neurol.* 2017;74:1223−1227.

25. Larsen P, Stoddart H, Griess M. Ophthalmoscopy using an eye simulator model. *Clin Teach.* 2014;11:99−103.

26. McMillan HJ, Writer H, Moreau KA, et al. Lumbar puncture simulation in pediatric residency training: improving procedural competence and decreasing anxiety. *BMC Med Educ.* 2016;16:198.

27. Richard S, Mione G, Varoqui C, et al. Simulation training for emergency teams to manage acute ischemic stroke by telemedicine. *Med Baltim.* 2016;95:e3924.

28. Lazzara EH, Benishek LE, Dietz AS, et al. Eight critical factors in creating and implementing a successful simulation program. *Jt Comm J Qual Patient Saf.* 2014;40:21−29.

CHAPTER 3

Developing Scenarios

Didactic lectures are part of hospital teaching and often come spontaneously for physicians with a high command of the topic. The traditional hospital teaching style of bedside instruction occurs whenever a resident or fellow presents a case to the attending physician. The senior physician guides the trainee during evaluation and management, tailoring their level of supervision to the learner's skill level. This impromptu method is established and almost universally practiced.

Simulation based teaching is very different: heavily scripted, meticulously prepared, and rehearsed. Any new scenario starts with an idea and ends with a fully elaborated, realistic clinical event. Ideas for a simulation scenario often come easily, but the workability requires innovative thinking and testing in a simulation center. Reports of mishaps or morbidity and mortality conferences may suggest ideas, but most currently used simulation scenarios are about recognizable, understandable, and manageable neurologic disorders and not the so-called "zebras" or unusual situations. The goal of scenario writing, therefore, is to create a believable environment; that is, avoid oversimplification and avoid overwhelming the learner with a host of complexities.

Neurology scenario writers should anticipate "neurophobia" (nonneurologists worried that they will be unqualified as a result of the nature of their specialty). Therefore, neurology-based scenarios should contain basic but essential knowledge for any physician involved in the care of patients with acute neurologic disease. The core of acute neurologic simulation scenarios best imitate emergency department and intensive care unit reality and, therefore, depends on what the writer of the scenario recalls of certain clinical situations. Ideally, writers should themselves be senior physicians, or senior, experienced physicians should serve as consultants to the writers. Many years of experience—and, specifically, years of witnessing missteps—facilitates the development of a simulation scenario.[1,2] In fact, much scenario writing involves thinking through the initial ambiguous presentation and maturation of the patient's problem and recreating that experience for the learner.

A scenario design begins by identifying a clinical challenge.[3] The challenge could involve recognition of imminent neuromuscular respiratory failure, recognition of a deteriorating patient with an acute brain lesion, recognition of aneurysmal subarachnoid hemorrhage, treatment of increased intracranial pressure, or treatment of status epilepticus. Once the topic is selected, the vignette outline is created, usually based on a remembered patient, which could be modified further with common pitfalls, "worst-case" scenarios, and traps. The scenario writer will then develop a narrative flow of the scenario including initial parameters, laboratory or ancillary testing, planned events, transitions, and response to anticipated interventions. To sustain the attention of the participants (i.e., learner, actors, and facilitator), most scenarios should be brief, which also allows the learner to go through a few in one session. This chapter discusses the methodology of scenario writing; additional assistance with design is available online.[4]

THE SCENARIOS
Designing Scenarios

It is useful initially to determine the level of complexity (Table 3.1). It is also important to distinguish between the primary goal, which is the main lesson to be learned, and secondary goals, which relate to management of the overwhelming information and how best to achieve good communication and professionalism. Simulation may expose the inability of some learners to do what they are expected to do. Any scenario should have some degree of flexibility (and fixes) when participants move in the wrong direction or do something unexpectedly. A learner can be given study material (i.e., guidelines, suggestions for book chapters) in the form of a list to prevent them from predicting the upcoming scenarios.

The best scenarios start with a so-called "case briefing," where the learner receives some information before the start of the scenario. This is usually a simple narrative about the patient. The idea here is to present the simulation in the same manner as a phone call or text page. The description should be relatively vague and open and should not contain the diagnosis or specific goal of the scenario. It should only provide basic information about the patient and the circumstances that brought the patient to the emergency

TABLE 3.1
Considerations in Scenario Design

	Key Feature	Goal	Example
Stressful	Emotion	Develop approach	Patient/family conflict
Complicated	Multiple choices	Prioritization	Unresponsive patient
Critical	Mistakes	Recognize error	Status epilepticus
Uncommon	Rare exposure	Refresher course	Brain death

department or the intensive care unit. The scenario should clearly identify the nature of the simulation room, whether it is an intensive care unit or emergency department, because in some scenarios, urgent triage is necessary before even continuing the scenario (for example, see Chapter 17, which discourages the performance of brain death determination examinations in the emergency department—when typically there is little reliable knowledge about the patient).

The scenario should have a clear description of the room setup and props needed, which may include medication infusions and IV fluids, but also tools required for examination of the simulated patient (Table 3.2). Scenarios in acute neurology also have the opportunity to use moulage, which is defined as an art that depicts illness and injury.

Scenarios ideally need to work out a strategy for when an unexpected course occurs; this is when learners completely deviate from the planned scenario and need redirection. Stopping the scenario is also an option if redirection cannot be achieved by the facilitator. This is the most difficult aspect of scenario design and requires that the scenario be modified after multiple trainings show where the scenario can possibly go wrong. It is important to avoid the "too much" scenario that quickly overwhelms the learner with lots of information, which creates a stressful situation and a poor experience for the learner. Scenarios can also be too fast-moving, in which time allowed for careful thinking and elaborating on the problem at hand is too short and the learner has no time to gather his or her thoughts. In general, it is also important to avoid scenarios in which the learner has to discover minute, easily overlooked details to solve the scenario, which may halt the normal flow. An example would be to leave multiple antidepressant drugs next to a simulated comatose patient—scenarios are not Sherlock Holmes mysteries.

TABLE 3.2
Common Setup Requirements

People needed	• Learner to be tested • Actors to play the patient or confederates (i.e., nurse, respiratory therapist, emergency medicine physician) • Instructor behind one-way mirror to facilitate
Equipment needed	• Mannequin • 2 headsets (confederate, facilitator) • Syringes • BP cuff • IV line and IV bags • Reflex hammer • Tuning fork • Laboratory results • Relevant imaging
Setup needed	• ED Face Sheet in folder attached to the door • Monitor showing changes in vital signs • Access to imaging • Phone line to instructor

Finally, the instructor may choose to use a rating form and questionnaire to obtain postexercise feedback from the learners. The questionnaire should collect information about the learner's experience. Some scenarios include an "automatic fail" point, where the scenario stops if the learner does not recognize an absolute critical point that must be resolved. This could be failure to diagnose the disorder or instituting inappropriate or inadequate treatments. In some situations, it might be useful to have potential future learners formulate their own learning objectives, which would improve responsiveness to the needs of the participant. These evaluation forms are often ad hoc, nonvalidated, and may change frequently, depending on the adjustments to the scenario. In most centers, fulfilling the preset key competencies should suffice, but debriefing faculty may decide to prioritize specific competencies (some competencies are obviously more important than others). Nevertheless, we have found that avoiding the pass/fail dichotomy and using the debriefing session to review each of the competencies is more worthwhile than assigning an artificial passing score.

The learner should be informed as to what is expected of them; some guidance is provided in Table 3.3. Actors do their best to mimic neurologic disease even if not all of them are "Oscar worthy." Employing a scenario that is "too easy" may cause the learner to feel insulted and not engaged. Learners should be informed that the scenario will not be graded and that individual results will be kept confidential. The learner's performance should never be discussed outside the simulation center, and confidentiality is emphasized and assumed between the trainees and instructors. Moreover, a single performance is a poor predictor of overall effectiveness. The debriefing should be done by experts in the field to avoid unnecessary hierarchy. In general, it is better to set up a scenario that can be used across specialties.

Scenarios are typically recorded, and learners cannot opt out of being recorded for educational purposes. The recording may be additionally useful for simulated patients, who can view and reflect on their performance. Participants should sign a release or consent to be filmed,

although the recording is eventually destroyed after debriefing unless it is in the context of research. It should also be emphasized to the participants that they may opt out of having their recording used for research.

Finally, the scenario will involve a number of embedded persons also known as "confederates." Each of their tasks can be written into the scenario. An important unresolved question is whether confederates may "ad lib" and how much improvisation is allowed. Generally, the responses of the confederates can be guided through headphones to facilitate creative adaptation to the unfolding situation. The ongoing intent is to guide the learner toward the set goal. Confederates can portray emergency department staff, nursing, or family members. When playing family members, confederates will have a set scenario and must stay "on script." Confederates playing an emergency department physician or nurse are given latitude to ask clarifying questions ("What exactly are you testing?" "What dose?" "What do you think is going on with this patient?") and may deviate slightly from the script as needed to improve the flow of the scenario. However, confederates should never deliberately mislead the learner or confuse the situation. Role-playing with professional actors in the simulation center differs from other techniques such as *role reversal* (the learner taking on the role of a difficult patient or family member) and *doubling* (participants stand behind a character and speak the thoughts, feelings, and attitude that they imagine the character might be thinking or feeling). Role-playing allows learners—in general—to find a treatment plan that is agreeable to the family and medically acceptable. Scenarios can involve a number of ethical and cultural conflicts and may concentrate on testing how to work through a situation where the family cannot let go. In other scenarios, they may find themselves telling family members their loved one has an irrecoverable brain injury or has died and is kept on artificial support.

Crafting Scenarios

The physician or healthcare worker that actually writes the scenario should oversee the full development of the scenario including directing and adapting it through trial and error. This is most important in developing role-playing, where character development (e.g., the difficult, intransigent family) is of utmost importance to make it believable and useful. Scenario writing is somewhat similar to writing a film script or play with emphasis on stage directions and dialog. Writing a scenario first requires deconstruction of the key competencies (Fig. 3.1). The scenario is made of several bits

TABLE 3.3
Instructions for Learners
• The actor or mannequin is mimicking a disorder that can evolve
• The actor is trying to portray neurologic disease and not a functional neurologic symptom or disorder
• Tests you ordered for the patient can be normal on purpose
• It is not about a good or bad experience—it is about the experience
• You are watched and videotaped
• Nobody should talk about your performance outside of the simulation center
• Do not apply pain stimuli to actors

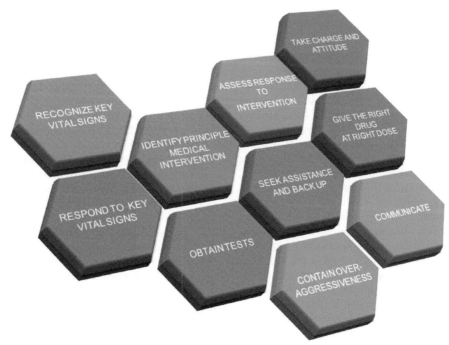

FIG. 3.1 Deconstructing the key competencies of a simulation scenario.

and pieces, and writers may have to go back to these main components. When crafting a scenario, writers may begin by trying to include "everything" but subsequently whittle it down to just the most essential problems. Each step must have a logical flow. Writers can only proceed with scripting after they have identified the reasons for teaching the neurologic emergency. How does it look to a learner when he steps into the room, and what kind of action should be taken? How does the learner take care of the patient? Does the learner get to the heart of the matter and fulfill the primary objective? How does the learner proceed, and do the interventions meet standard of care? How does the learner seek information and communicate?

Consider 10 steps with writing scenarios

Step 1—Decide what you want to teach but keep your audience in mind: basic scenarios for novice learners; specialized scenarios for advanced learners.

Step 2—Identify 10 or fewer key competencies. In other words, what are the most important things to know to manage the presented clinical situation? The ideal learner (1) recognizes the disorder, (2) anticipates its clinical course, (3) initiates search for causes or contributing factors, (4) addresses code status, (5) uses appropriate dose of medication,

(6) appropriately manages deteriorating vital signs, (7) requests appropriate diagnostic tests, (8) correctly interprets test results, (9) stabilizes the patient and treats the disorder, and (10) appropriately explains decisions and communicates with family.

Step 3—Create a vignette (choose age, gender, relevant past medical history, and what brought them into the emergency department or intensive care unit).

Step 4—Develop the learning objectives; these will necessarily include the key competencies required to manage the clinical situation presented but should also be broader in scope, and inclusive of the entire fund of knowledge necessary to care for any patient with the same pathology.

Step 5—Write a natural flow of the scenario. Start with the moment the learner enters the room and is handed the patient's face sheet. When writing the flow, it is easiest first to envision the right way to do things. While doing so, try to imagine how a learner would interact with the mannequin or simulated patient.

Step 6—Identify common missteps, and write down how to deal with them when they occur in simulation. Do not allow too much improvisation. It is also helpful to suggest ways to challenge more advanced learners and to adapt the scenario for different types of learners.

Step 7—Bring the case to life by writing scripts for the confederate and other personnel including careful stage direction of how to portray neurologic findings.

Step 8—Practice "dry runs" of the scenario. Scripts must be easily understandable instructions devoid of medical jargon, given that the simulation staff may include people with no medical background.

Step 9—Develop a clear approach to the debriefing session. The debriefing is not only used to review the scenario but also to fill in the gaps to ensure the learning objectives are met.

Step 10—Finally, inform the simulation center which materials have to be available and which personnel are required.

Following development of a scenario, it should be piloted to collect and analyze learner feedback, to note criticisms, and ultimately, to make adjustments.

Rehearsing Scenarios

Rehearsals often lead to a rewrite. It quickly becomes clear what portions of the scenario lack credibility and which are too complicated for the learner to recognize or treat. Simple adjustments may suffice, but some parts, particularly those requiring "on the fly" adjustments by the facilitator behind the one-way mirror, may require better, more detailed scripting. Once the scenario is well developed and completed on paper, a "read-through" follows. This session brings together all participants (except the learner) to analyze each step of the exercise. Instructions for confederates and actors are shown in Tables 3.4 and 3.5.

First, participants discuss an ideal scenario and the sequence of events. Most confederates and instructors are passive observers except for guiding the learner with simple cues. Free communication with the facilitator is important but may lead to confusion. It is better to have a clear sense of how to communicate and, particularly, at which time points in the scenario. Practicing the scenario also allows identification and refinement of facilitator cues. These include inconspicuous foot taps, which the actor understands as a signal to change the presentation (e.g., demonstrate a seizure or new thunderclap headache). Clear directives should be discussed, although the facilitator behind the one-way screen may allow some improvisation to respond to various learner decisions and behaviors. Single scenarios may have more than one acceptable course of action, so the facilitator must be flexible and allow the case to develop to its natural completion when

TABLE 3.4 Instructions for Actors
• Practice until confident in the script
• Try to imagine how the patient would feel
• Try to focus on a few important clinical signs
• Be educated about the simulated disorder
• Identify potential barriers and request clarification from the facilitator
• Review predetermined cues from facilitator

TABLE 3.5 Instructions for Confederates
• This is a realistic drama - do not overact
• Understand context of the scenario
• Strive for conventionality
• Develop a good audio rapport with the instructor via the headsets
• Remain sympathetic
• Increase learners' engagement
• Help to move the flow of the scenario forward but do not cue learners without prompting from the facilitator

possible. As long as the learning objectives are met, the scenario is successful in achieving its goal. Some learners will get to the heart of the problem quickly; others, more slowly and with detours. A few will never get there—causing the scenario to stop prematurely.

Second, a dress rehearsal should be carried out with a learner who will not participate in future scenarios. This dry run is crucial and may even prompt a major revision if the run-through exposes significant flaws. Often, the revisions are simplifications. Although it should closely approximate actual clinical situations, actors in these role-play exercises have an opportunity to confront the learner (e.g., unpredictability of responses by family members), which may push learners out of their comfort zones. In developing these complex scenarios, an improvisational, spontaneous scenario could lead to further development of a script, but major deviations from the script should only be for a rehearsal. We have found that things get better over time once a workable "flow" is established.[5-14]

Writing scenarios designed to teach medical communication skills requires more detail because a character is being developed and the actor must be able to embody the character and portray a specific personality, mood, or stance. Many interactions of families and physicians are quite predictable and repeatedly heard in family conferences, and each of them can be written in a scenario or at least discussed "he would never want to be a vegetable," and "I have heard of patients coming out of coma doing very well"). Actors should avoid a highly stylized performance, but several important and commonly employed coping mechanisms are potentially useful for training. These are (1) intellectualization with laser focus on laboratory values or vital signs taken out of context to avoid emotional acceptance of the big picture, (2) denial while holding out for a miracle, (3) passive aggression (the socially acceptable response to feelings of aggression) manifested by sarcasm, distrust, and negativism, and (4) avoidance (the easygoing-but-indecisive procrastinator). This character development may also use gesticulation and a certain voice volume. The raising of an eyebrow, the rolling of eyes, a shout, and a whisper can all contribute to a sophisticated role-playing scenario. Yelling or "flipping out" occur occasionally during family conferences and can be allowed if the goal is to stun the learner. Generally, it is better to tone down overbearing actors and to keep a realistic perspective. Role-play could potentially include cultural issues such as ethnic customs and religious practices, particularly as they might affect attitudes regarding delivery of bad news, withdrawal of support, or organ donation.

CONCLUSIONS

Simulation of a neurologic emergency in progress requires a script with detailed dialogs and instructions. Scenario writing must be succinct and straightforward. Generally, it is better to be all-inclusive initially and gradually eliminate unworkable ideas. There are some simple conventions. The objectives should (1) correspond to the expertise and level of the learner, (2) fit with the expected outcome, (3) be based on best (ideally evidence-based) knowledge and standard of care, (4) be achievable in a short timeframe, and (5) result in a good overall learning experience. Developing scenarios for role-playing in acute neurologic

conditions requires significant detail and preparatory work to build a useful setup. Most scenarios mature over time; some may not make a second version and stall. This book describes scenarios that have worked in our simulation center and that we believe are fully transferable.

REFERENCES

1. Blum RH, et al. Simulation-based assessment to reliably identify key resident performance attributes. *Anesthesiology.* 2018;128:821−831.
2. Gaba DM, et al. Simulation-based training in anesthesia crisis resource management (ACRM): a decade of experience. *Simul Gaming.* 2001;32:175−193.
3. Bambini D. Writing a simulation scenario: a step-by-step guide. *AACN Adv Crit Care.* 2016;27:62−70.
4. S.I.R.C. *The Simulation Design Website;* 2009. Available from: http://sirc.nln.org/mod/forum/discuss.php?d=83.
5. Karam VY, Hanane Barakat H, Aouad M, et al. Effect of a simulation-based workshop on breaking bad news for anesthesiology residents: an intervention study. *BMC Anesthesiol.* 2017;17:77.
6. Harden R. Twelve tips on teaching and learning how to break bad news. *Med Teach.* 1996;18:275−278.
7. Watling C, Brown J. Education research: communication skills for neurology residents-structured teaching and reflective practice. *Neurology.* 2007;69:22.
8. Rosenbaum M, Ferguson K, Lobas J. Teaching medical students and residents skills for delivering bad news: a review of strategies. *Acad Med.* 2004;79:107−117.
9. Bowyer M, Rawn L, Hanson J, et al. Combining high-fidelity human patient simulators with a standardized family member: a novel approach to teaching breaking bad news. *Stud Health Technol Inf.* 2006;119:67−72.
10. Azoulay E, Chevret S, Leleu G, et al. Half the families of intensive care unit patients experience inadequate communication with physicians. *Crit Care Med.* 2000;28: 3044−3049.
11. Skye EP, Wagenschutz H, Steiger JA, Kumagai AK. Use of interactive theater and role play to develop medical students' skills in breaking bad news. *Cancer Educ.* 2014;29: 704−708.
12. Maynard DW. Delivering bad news in emergency care medicine. *Acute Med Surg.* 2016;4:3−11.
13. Baile WF1, Blatner A. Teaching communication skills: using action methods to enhance role-play in problem-based learning. *Simul Health.* 2014;9:220−227.
14. Maguire P, Pitceathly C. Key communication skills and how to acquire them. *BMJ.* 2002;325:697.

CHAPTER 4

Simulating Traumatic Brain Injury

Traumatic brain injury (TBI) is seen by multiple disciplines, often starting in the emergency department, and its presentation to emergency departments can trigger involvement of trauma surgeons, neurosurgeons, and neurointensivists. Priorities of care are determined by the type and severity of injury and cause of the decline in vital signs.

Simulation in trauma—polytrauma in particular—is well established as an educational model, and current simulation centers are offering sophisticated scenarios for training. Healthcare worker from multiple disciplines have gone through these training sessions, which have led to improved knowledge and skills in team management of any type of severe trauma.[1] As most previous simulation studies have discovered, training of trauma teams using simulation improves most learners' ability to recognize the need for procedures and hones the skills necessary to perform these procedures, but there is yet no evidence to support improvement in clinical parameters.[2] Most evaluations of simulation of trauma have only shown that simulation scenarios can improve teamwork coordination, which could theoretically help the patient.[3,4] Experience on simulating TBI and using brain-protection strategies could be further developed.

Management of TBI has multiple tiers and goals that must be achieved within the first 12 h.[5,6] The principles of early management of TBI in the emergency department remain fairly established, and regularly revised guidelines have been proposed by multiple organizations.[7,8] These guidelines—providing the necessities of brain protection—can readily be a basis for scenario development. In this chapter, we describe a simulation scenario that highlights the initial management, correction of vital signs, and reasoned approach to increased intracranial pressure.

THE PROBLEM BEFORE US

TBI can occur in the setting of polytrauma or in isolation. Both are equally important, but TBI is often overshadowed by polytrauma and emergent surgical interventions needed to, frankly, save the patient's life.

Often, assessment will have already begun in the field at the site of the accident. There, acute management of TBI is initially performed by paramedic units. Severe trauma is always anticipated, particularly if the patient has been extracted from a serious car wreck.

Many patients with severe TBI come to the emergency department with a decreased level of consciousness or deteriorate soon after arrival (the so-called "walk, talk, and deteriorate" category). For attending physicians, it is important to realize immediately that no patient with TBI is truly stable or, indeed, anything less than serious and that the clinical situation can change rapidly from problems that lay in store.

In the ED, the initial assessment of the patient is usually done using the Glasgow Coma Scale (GCS), which is helpful for triage and estimation of the need for intubation (i.e., GCS <8 = intubate!). However, once in the hospital, this scale is nothing more than an approximation of the neurologic examination, and important findings (i.e., localizing signs, brainstem reflexes) are not measured with this scale. Most of the numerical scores used in conversation are not much better than designating the patient alert (GCS, 15), drowsy (GCS, 10−14), or comatose (GCS, <8). A full neurologic and neurosurgical assessment is needed to document the clinical condition at the moment of arrival.

Next, for both the neurointensivist and neurosurgeon, it is important to have immediate, detailed knowledge of CT scan abnormalities in the setting of trauma. Abnormalities requiring immediate attention include lobar contusions, acute subdural hematomas, or even more urgent epidural hematomas. Brain contusions can blossom quickly and change a patient's neurologic status in a matter of hours. Diffuse, traumatic subarachnoid hemorrhage is significant and may indicate brain contusions may be seen on a follow-up CT scan. The CT scan must be reviewed to assess the probability of increased intracranial pressure, judged by evidence of early cerebral edema or mass effect. Increased intracranial pressure can be assumed when the basal cisterns are effaced and ventricles are slit-like. Any patient that looks worse than the CT scan suggests could have an additional factor playing a major role, and in most emergency departments, this could point toward a confounding intoxication, anoxic-ischemic injury or a major abnormality in a vital sign—profound hypoxemia or shock.

Many level I trauma centers have defined the initial management of TBI but guidelines also have identified deficiencies in evidence and glaring gaps in understanding of mechanisms.[7]

Blood pressure and adequate oxygenation need to be ensured, and patients should receive hyperosmolar therapy and hyperventilation if there is presumed evidence of increased intracranial pressure (ICP). Measurement of increased ICP and cerebral perfusion pressure is not possible or feasible in the emergency department (and even in some ICUs) and therefore becomes more of an issue after the patient is later admitted to a neuro-science intensive care unit. Furthermore, there have been important recommendations on the use of anes-thetics, corticosteroids, and aggressive methods of pro-phylaxis.[7] Each can be built into a simulation scenario.

Many experts in the field have participated in identi-fying the best approaches to improve clinical care and research. The current issues are classification of TBI types and severity, use of biomarkers, further research in the usefulness of advanced MRI methods, and value of new brain-monitoring technology, all of which could provide a better understanding of the mechanisms of TBI.[9,10] Furthermore, assessment of outcome of TBI is relevant, but current metrics are limited, and there is a need for better outcome assessment and prognostic modeling. Most importantly, better ways of organizing systems of care are needed throughout the world.[9] Despite these shortcomings, there is reasonable empiric evidence on how best to approach and manage patients with TBI.

Once the patient arrives at the emergency depart-ment, an ABCDE trauma evaluation is often used, which guides all healthcare workers through a system-atic approach. The components of ABCDE are shown in Fig. 4.1. Simple in concept, it provides some safe-guards on how to think through these complex presen-tations, but ABCDE method undervalues assessment of the brain.

There are several initial considerations when dealing with a patient with TBI. A step-by-step approach ensures "covering of the basics" and is helpful for any physician in the emergency department asking "what do I do now?"[11]

The management of increased ICP, in general, in-volves placing the head of the bed at 30 degrees, brief hyperventilation to $PaCO_2$ of 30–35 mmHg, and use of osmotic agents (in most cases beginning with

Basics of the ABCDE Approach

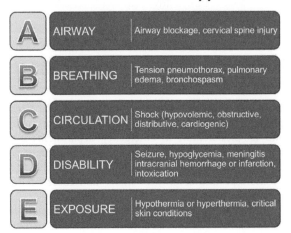

FIG. 4.1   ABCDE of trauma.

mannitol, 25%, 1–2 g/kg, or hypertonic saline, usually 30 cc of 23.4% NaCl). Induced hypothermia is ineffec-tive and could potentially worsen outcome. It is un-known whether prewarming of a mildly hypothermic patient improves outcome.

Next, the CT scan should indicate whether neurosur-gical intervention is needed for a traumatic brain contu-sion with mass effect. Decisions are also guided by the neurologic examination, but large contusions causing mass effect need evacuation unless the exam is very poor (i.e., loss of multiple brainstem reflexes). Before surgery —and certainly if the patient has been trans-ferred from another hospital—a repeat CT scan is required to assess the brain tissue shift or whether there is growth of contusional volume. Management of pene-trating injury is rarely neurosurgical and certainly not when there is a trajectory through both hemispheres and when the diencephalic structures and mesenceph-alon are destroyed. Surgeons usually consider removal of bone and bullet fragments in patients with little or any preservation of consciousness. Gunshots may also lacerate important arteries including the vertebral artery with gunshots through the oropharynx. The presence of an epidural hematoma (a rapidly growing arterial bleed) invariably results in a neurosurgical evacuation. Outcome is strongly influenced by whether there is obliteration of the basal cisterns and whether there is a brain tissue shift. Surgery for acute subdural hematoma (a mostly slow-growing venous bleed on admission CT scan) is considered if the subdural hematoma has a thickness greater than 1 cm or midline shift of more than 5 mm on CT scan. Large subdural hematomas presenting in the absence of many brain-stem reflexes, particularly both pupil and corneal reflexes, will likely not result in improved outcome after evacuation. However, fixed, dilated pupils alone should not necessarily dissuade a neurosurgeon from proceeding with the evacuation.

In addition, one should always consider associated spinal cord injury and manage accordingly. A cervical collar should be in place. Full cervical spine X-rays and, preferably, multiplanar CT are needed in any patient with TBI and fall—even from standing height. Ligamentous injuries at the craniocervical junction are often associated with high-energy trauma, but odontoid fractures are also easily missed. Spinal fractures require a multidisciplinary response, often with input from a spine surgeon. With evidence of possible neck trauma, physicians should consider traumatic vascular injury. Dissecting injury to the carotid and vertebral arteries may lead to acute occlusion of the dissected artery and, depending on available compensatory collaterals, may lead to an ischemic stroke. This complication of the trauma may only become apparent on repeat CT scans.

Second, it is important to support the vital signs, appreciate subtle changes or trends, and start intracranial hypertension management early. Acute hypoxemia or persistent hypotension may cause additional anoxic-ischemic injury, and these abnormalities are often not well recognized during transportation of the patient. However, there is no proven benefit from temperature lowering or hypothermia.[12–14] Failure to aggressively control ICP is common and, particularly in the first hours, could lead to early secondary brainstem injury. Elevation of the head of the bed, hyperventilation, and hyperosmolar therapy are the first interventions.[15,16] Neurosurgeons have noted that in many patients with refractory increased ICP, decompressive craniectomy may not only facilitate management of intracranial hypertension, but may affect outcome in some patients. Decompressive surgery is often an adequate treatment for refractory increased intracranial pressure, and the threshold to proceed with this procedure should be generally low.[17–19] Neurosurgeons often do not replace a bone flap after evacuation of a traumatic contusion or large subdural hematoma in anticipation of postoperative swelling. Finally, the patient may need placement of an intracranial pressure monitoring device. Mostly this is placed in the ICU, but may also be placed during surgery to evacuate a contusion or hematoma.[20,21] The indications for ICP monitor placement are coma and evidence of diffuse cerebral edema as indicated by obliteration of ventricles or small compressed ventricles.

THE PRESENTING CLINICAL PROBLEM

The patient presented here is a 54-year-old male who was in a motor vehicle accident but never lost consciousness. He has been unattended for some time, but there were no serious worrisome vital-sign abnormalities. The vital signs show mild hypotension and mild hypoxemia. The learner has the opportunity to request imaging studies, including a CT scan, chest X-ray, and cervical spine X-ray, all of which are available in the room. The main objectives of this simulation scenario are shown in Table 4.1.

The SBAR technique can be a useful tool in communication of conditions requiring acute triage (SBAR is an acronym for Situation, Background, Assessment, and Recommendation).

Preparation

The scenario uses SimMan 3G. A voiceover is used. The monitor shows a blood pressure of 90/50 mmHg, normal heart and respiratory rates, oxygen saturation of 90%, and normal temperature of 36.5°C. The key competences are shown in Fig. 4.2. This scenario works through a combination of treating abnormal signs and treating increased intracranial pressure. The scenario setup is detailed in Table 4.2.

Coaching Actors

Depending on the desired objectives, a full trauma level I team can be simulated, but we concentrate on isolated TBI. This scenario is best simplified by having one nurse or an ED physician as the confederate. Instructions are shown in Table 4.3.

THE IDEAL LEARNER

L enters the emergency department and is provided with a brief history of the patient. The *CONF* portraying the

---

TABLE 4.1
Objectives

- Considers possibility of spinal cord injury
- Places head at 30 degrees
- Ensures adequate blood pressure, oxygen saturation, and coagulation
- Interprets CT of the brain and plans repeat imaging
- Manages intracranial hypertension effectively (brief hyperventilation, considers comorbidities in selection of hyperosmolar therapy, uses proper doses of drugs)
- Considers prophylactic antiseizure drugs
- Consults neurosurgery

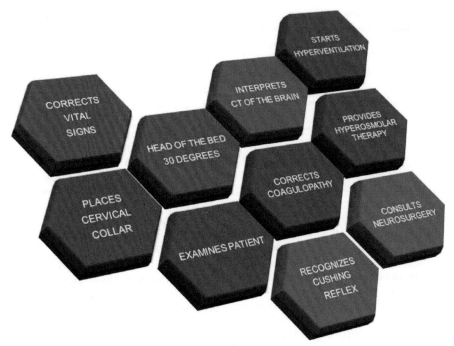

FIG. 4.2 Deconstructing key competencies in traumatic brain injury.

emergency room nurse will say, "This patient was found after a motor vehicle accident. He is mildly hypothermic and has normal vital signs. The trauma likely involved a car rollover. The trauma surgeon signed off and believes most of it is medical management of TBI. He had a pulmonary embolus 6 months ago but we do not know much more."

Detailed neurologic examination on SimMan 3G is not possible, but L immediately identifies pupillary light reflexes and absent motor responses to pain. When questions are asked, P (in a voiceover by the facilitator) is confused. Noting that P is mildly hypotensive and hypoxemic, L administers additional fluids (500 cc) and increases the fraction of inspired oxygen on the ventilator. L then requests that $CONF$ place a cervical collar and elevate the head of bed to 30 degrees. L asks for laboratory tests including chemistry, complete blood count, and coagulation studies as well as a chest x-ray and both head and cervical spine CT scans. $CONF$ provides the laboratory results and directs L to the CT scan (Fig. 4.3). Noting an INR of 2.8, normal sodium, normal glucose, and bifrontal contusions with surrounding edema, L immediately requests administration of a single dose of prothrombin complex concentrate and 10 mg IV vitamin K. $CONF$ then asks for further direction ("what else needs to be done?" "where should he be admitted—

to the neurosciences ICU or the trauma ICU?") L first confirms normalization of blood pressure and oxygen saturation, and noting a BP of 110/80 mmHg and oxygen saturation of 98%, asks to speak to the trauma surgeon who evaluated P and requests neurosurgical evaluation in the ED.

While deliberation on appropriate triage is taking place, the facilitator increases the blood pressure to 200/120 mmHg, lowers the heart rate to 50 bpm, and makes the pupils nonreactive to light. $CONF$ alerts L to the changes, and in response, he reexamines P. Finding the pupils to be fixed and dilated and interpreting the clinical changes to be reflective of a Cushing reflex, L administers 1 g/kg mannitol or 30 cc of 23.4% saline. He adjusts the ventilator settings to achieve minute ventilation sufficient to obtain a PCO_2 in the 30s, asks that neurosurgery be called emergently, and orders a new stat CT scan. When asked by $CONF$ if dexamethasone should be given, L resists its administration. On reevaluation of the patient, the pupils are again reactive to light. When neurosurgery calls back (facilitator via a direct line in the room), L uses SBAR technique to communicate the situation, background, his assessment of increased ICP and tissue shift, and recommendation of assessment for surgical options. Simulation ends.

TABLE 4.2
Scenario Setup for Traumatic Brain Injury

People needed	• Actor to play nurse or ED physician • Attending physician or neurocritical care fellow to facilitate
Equipment needed	• Simulation mannequin • Syringes • Mechanical ventilator • BP cuff • IV lines • Oxygen by nasal cannula • Laboratory results • Cervical collar
Setup needed	• Reactive pupils • BP 90/50 mmHg • SPO$_2$ 90% • Temperature 36.5°C • Head CT on monitor (monitor turned off until learner requests imaging); X-ray of chest and CT of cervical spine available

TABLE 4.3
Actor Instructions before Simulation

- SimMan 3G as simulated patient using SimMan voice module (Instructor provides inconclusive answers such as "I don't know," "Where am I?" or, "Yeah?")
- Confederate attends to requests (labs, neuroimaging)
- Confederate conveys uncertainty about management; professes him/herself to be more familiar with general trauma
- Confederate sets tone for a rushed environment ("other patients need to be seen")
- Confederate asks about priorities, blood pressure goals, consults required before admission, and admission location

THE NOT-SO-IDEAL LEARNER

Major difficulties with recognition of the severity of traumatic injury have been detected during our sessions. The following errors in judgment have been made.

1. *The learner does not secure cervical spine or obtain spinal imaging.* Any trauma (including fall from standing height) with a decreased level of consciousness should assume injury to the spine and a collar should be placed automatically. A normal CT spine does not exclude spine instability and requires a clinical examination and, if that is not possible, an MRI of the spine.

2. *The learner does not use adequate measures to reduce ICP.* The learner does not provide hyperventilation or mannitol or does not place the head of the bed at 30 degrees. Each learner should, almost reflexively, start with this combination of interventions. Some immediately request hypertonic saline, which cannot be easily used because it needs central access. By failing to recognize this, the learner could cause significant phlebitis. Even acute access to a femoral vein (so called "direct fem stick") may not be fully safe and should only be used to prevent terminal brainstem injury from shift. Learners need to know how to provide hyperventilation (mostly by increasing rate rather than tidal volume) and where to target the PaCO$_2$.

3. *The learner does not appreciate the severity of frontal lobe contusions.* Many frontal contusions cause more mass effect, which may precipitously increase ICP causing both a surge in blood pressure and bradycardia (Cushing reflex). Although these contusions may seem trivial, they are associated with a high likelihood of clinical worsening. Frontal contusions are frequently the culprit when patients seem reasonably well on initial presentation and then worsen. Often more contusions are present at other sites not initially visualized on the CT scan.

4. *The learner does not optimize vital signs.* Corrections should include improvement of blood pressure parameters and avoidance of hypoxemia. This is often recognized early by ED or trauma specialists, but learners in the neurology or neurosurgery specialties tend to recognize it late.

5. *The learner fails to appreciate need to correct anticoagulation.* The elevated INR can contribute to expansion of the hematoma. In this situation, one dose of prothrombin complex concentrate is likely sufficient in combination with IV vitamin K. A repeat INR should be checked 30 min after the administration to prove coagulopathy reversal.

ADAPTING THE SCENARIO

The scenario can be adapted for traumatic head injury by adding a brief seizure, which would add the need for antiseizure drugs. The instructor can further manipulate the vital signs to indicate that the patient might have internal bleeding elsewhere that indicates a polytrauma rather than purely traumatic brain or spine injury. Further adjustments can be made to teach

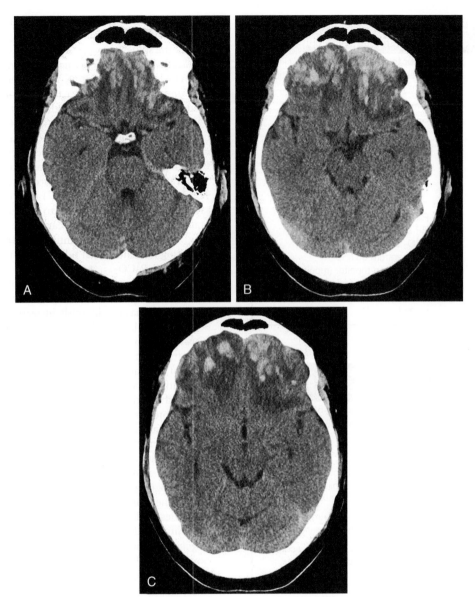

FIG. 4.3 Frontal lobe contusions on admission CT.

that attention to hypovolemic shock—while important—may also lead to failure to recognize and treat TBI.

Care should be taken when adding complexity to this particular scenario. It should not replace a full level I trauma team scenario in which learners must take charge of polytrauma. In general, it is better not to add a number of systemic complications that could overwhelm the learner, who likely is not a trauma surgeon. However, possible adjustments to the scenario include (1) blood loss and hypotension prompting blood transfusion or (2) lung contusion prompting increased PEEP ventilation and increased F_1O_2. Opportunities to practice placement of an ICP monitor or ventriculostomy using simulation are not widely available and should be developed.

TABLE 4.4
Guidelines for the Management of Severe Traumatic Brain Injury[7]

Blood pressure	• SBP ≥ 100 mmHg • PaO₂ > 60 mml Ig • SPO₂ > 90%
Threshold for intracranial pressure (ICP)	• ICP < 22 mmHg
Threshold for cerebral perfusion pressure (CPP)	• CPP 60–70 mmHg
Hyperosmolar therapy	• Mannitol, 0.5–2 g/kg body weight
Hyperventilation	• PCO₂ ≤ 25 mg not recommended as prophylaxis • Avoid first 24 h after injury • Use only as temporary measure
Anesthetics	• Barbiturates not recommended • Caution with propofol
Corticosteroids	• Corticosteroids are not recommended
Prophylaxis	• Early tracheostomy • Heparin to prevent venous thromboembolic disease (or vena cava filter) • Antiseizure prophylaxis recommended for up to 1 week to reduce incidence of early seizures • Antiseizure prophylaxis not recommended for preventing late seizures

DEBRIEFING

The debriefing reviews the major objectives and includes the classification of TBI and important subtypes. Review of the causes of deterioration in the emergency department is important because they may not be readily known. The potential for additional intoxication and its effect on neurologic examination can be discussed. Methods to stabilize the patient's vital signs and cervical spine, manage intracranial hypertension, interpret the CT scan, and respond accordingly are all discussed in detail. The main goals of brain resuscitation are an important discussion point, and each parameter is an opportunity for further elaboration (e.g., "How does mannitol work?" "How do we measure adequate control of ICP and how do we dose osmotic agents?" "What are the complications of hyperosmolar therapy?" "Who is at greatest risk of deterioration?" "What are the clinical signs of increased ICP, mass effect and brain tissue shift?") The main consensus statements of the TBI guidelines as shown in Table 4.4 can be discussed.

CONCLUSIONS

Simulation of TBI is feasible and necessary because it addresses a number of important decision points in acute brain injury. Decisions not only include judging the severity and type of head injury but also assessment of fractures elsewhere and preventive measures such as placement of the cervical collar. It provides an opportunity to discuss the fundamentals of intracranial hypertension management that include initiation of hyperventilation, hyperosmolar therapy, and maintenance of cerebral perfusion pressure, largely by supporting the systemic blood pressure. The indications for neurosurgical intervention, particularly removal of contusions or decompressive craniectomy as a last resort to treat refractory ICP, can be taught.

REFERENCES

1. Gjeraa K, Moller TP, Ostergaard D. Efficacy of simulation-based trauma team training of non-technical skills. A systematic review. *Acta Anaesthesiol Scand.* 2014;58: 775–787.
2. Capella J, Smith S, Philp A, et al. Teamwork training improves the clinical care of trauma patients. *J Surg Educ.* 2010;67:439–443.
3. Shapiro MJ, Morey JC, Small SD, et al. Simulation based teamwork training for emergency department staff: does it improve clinical team performance when added to an existing didactic teamwork curriculum? *Qual Saf Health Care.* 2004;13:417–421.
4. Steinemann S, Berg B, Skinner A, et al. In situ, multidisciplinary, simulation-based teamwork training improves early trauma care. *J Surg Educ.* 2011;68:472–477.
5. Garvin R, Mangat HS. Emergency neurological life support: severe traumatic brain injury. *Neurocrit Care.* 2017; 27:159–169.
6. Abou El Fadl MH, O'Phelan KH. Management of traumatic brain injury: an update. *Neurosurg Clin N Am.* 2018;29: 213–221.

7. Carney N, Totten AM, O'Reilly C, et al. Guidelines for the management of severe traumatic brain injury, fourth edition. *Neurosurgery*. 2017;80:6−15.

8. Geeraerts T, Le Guen M. Checklists and cognitive aids in simulation training and daily critical care practice: simple tools to improve medical performance and patient outcome. *Anaesth Crit Care Pain Med*. 2018;37:3−4.

9. Maas AIR, Menon DK, Adelson PD, et al. Traumatic brain injury: integrated approaches to improve prevention, clinical care, and research. *Lancet Neurol*. 2017;16:987−1048.

10. Werner C, Engelhard K. Pathophysiology of traumatic brain injury. *Br J Anaesth*. 2007;99:4−9.

11. Wijdicks EFM, Rabinstein AA, Hocker SE, et al. Neurocritical Care: What Do I Do Now? In: *What Do I Do Now*. 2nd ed. New York: Oxford University Press; 2016:336.

12. Andrews PJ, Sinclair HL, Rodriguez A, et al. Hypothermia for intracranial hypertension after traumatic brain injury. *N Engl J Med*. 2015;373:2403−2412.

13. Clifton GL, Miller ER, Choi SC, et al. Lack of effect of induction of hypothermia after acute brain injury. *N Engl J Med*. 2001;344:556−563.

14. Sydenham E, Roberts I, Alderson P. Hypothermia for traumatic head injury. *Cochrane Database Syst Rev*. 2009 Apr 15;(2):CD001048.

15. Cottenceau V, Masson F, Mahamid E, et al. Comparison of effects of equiosmolar doses of mannitol and hypertonic saline on cerebral blood flow and metabolism in traumatic brain injury. *J Neurotrauma*. 2011;28:2003−2012.

16. Rickard AC, Smith JE, Newell P, et al. Salt or sugar for your injured brain? A meta-analysis of randomised controlled trials of mannitol versus hypertonic sodium solutions to manage raised intracranial pressure in traumatic brain injury. *Emerg Med J*. 2014;31:679−683.

17. Cooper DJ, Rosenfeld JV, Murray L, et al. Decompressive craniectomy in diffuse traumatic brain injury. *N Engl J Med*. 2011;364:1493−1502.

18. Sahuquillo J, Arikan F. Decompressive craniectomy for the treatment of refractory high intracranial pressure in traumatic brain injury. *Cochrane Database Syst Rev*. 2006 Jan 25;(1):CD003983.

19. Shutter LA, Timmons SD. Intracranial pressure rescued by decompressive surgery after traumatic brain injury. *N Engl J Med*. 2016;375:1183−1184.

20. Alali AS, Fowler RA, Mainprize TG, et al. Intracranial pressure monitoring in severe traumatic brain injury: results from the American College of Surgeons Trauma Quality Improvement Program. *J Neurotrauma*. 2013;30:1737−1746.

21. Chesnut RM, Temkin N, Carney N, et al. A trial of intracranial-pressure monitoring in traumatic brain injury. *N Engl J Med*. 2012;367:2471−2481.

CHAPTER 5

Simulating Acute Carotid Artery Occlusion

Care of a patient with an ischemic stroke is an emergency and calls for action. Medical centers throughout the world have introduced "stroke alerts"—a page or text to a number of healthcare workers including pharmacists, phlebotomists, radiology technicians, stroke neurologists, and emergency department staff. With this alert comes a series of interventions and tests following a predetermined workflow. Time to intervention has become an obsession and for a good reason given that with each passing minute, eloquent neurons are lost. Central to this acute intervention are thrombolytics—currently predominantly tissue-type plasminogen activator (tPA)—and mechanical thrombectomy—with a stent retriever, aspiration catheter, or both—and they are proven interventions for select patients with acute ischemic stroke (Class I, evidence-based recommendation from the American Heart Association/American Stroke Association).[1]

The use of practiced protocols reduces the time to treatment.[2–4] The therapeutic benefit of tPA is greatest when given early and declines with time and there is no demonstrable benefit after 4.5 h.[5–8] Similarly, time from symptom onset to reperfusion with endovascular therapies correlates with clinical outcomes.[9,10] Best practices for reducing treatment times have been, and are being, evaluated and have led to adjustments in stroke protocols.[11,12]

Stroke simulation training has been shown to reduce tPA door-to-needle times in clinical practice.[13] Merely because stroke care has become tricky and risky, simulation of large territorial hemispheric acute ischemic stroke with all its immediate consequences offers an additional opportunity for learners to gain confidence in the skills required for rapid stroke assessment and management. Therefore, we have included this neuroemergency as a topic for simulation.

THE PROBLEM BEFORE US

Acute ischemic stroke with major initial neurologic deficit often involves an embolus lodged in the carotid or middle cerebral artery. These proximally located occlusions resolve with IV tPA alone in roughly one in 10 instances.[14] In other types of strokes with more downstream arterial occlusions, IV tPA improves the rate and speed of return to independent ambulation.[15] Endovascular treatment (if feasible—and then with only a small core of established infarct on neuroimaging) will therefore have to be considered and may still be successful even when the window of treatment is extended to 24 h from onset.[16,17] The endovascular treatment of stroke is a paradigm shift in acute stroke management, and results have been dramatic and, for some, produce immediate improvement in the angiogram suite.

The first priority in acute ischemic stroke is to obtain a focused history including a clear "last-known normal time" and to determine treatment eligibility. In patients who awaken from sleep with symptoms or are aphasic with an unwitnessed onset of symptoms, physicians must rely on the time the patient was last known to be without apparent neurologic deficits. This time point remains an important inclusion criterion for treatment with both tPA and mechanical clot retrieval. Administration of tPA is recommended within 4.5 h of symptom onset for patients meeting inclusion and exclusion criteria, and mechanical clot retrieval is recommended for select patients up to 24 h after "last-known normal time."[1]

The next step is to score the National Institutes of Health Stroke Scale (NIHSS). In acute ischemic stroke, the NIHSS is used to predict whether a large-vessel occlusion amenable to clot retrieval may be present. Specific NIHSS scores are also incorporated into inclusion and exclusion criteria for treatment decisions.[1] Physicians involved in the assessment and treatment of acute ischemic stroke as a regulatory measure now have to be competent in this skill but should also recognize its limitations in recognition of clinical signs of arterial occlusions in the posterior circulation (Chapter 6). Moreover, the total NIHSS score—particularly in the low ranges—may not always reflect the degree of disability.

A noncontrast head computed tomography (CT) scan should be performed within minutes of arrival to the emergency department (ED).[1] If the NIHSS is ≥6, CT angiogram (CTA) of the head and neck should also be performed at the time of the CT scan because the pretest probability of a large-vessel occlusion is higher and thus indicates potential for mechanical thrombectomy. Select patients presenting between 6 and 24 h of last-known normal time should also undergo CT perfusion at the time of the initial imaging.[1] CT perfusion series include cerebral blood volume (CBV), cerebral blood flow (CBF), and mean transit time (MTT). A matched perfusion abnormality between CBF and MTT or CBV maps strongly indicates nonsalvageable brain tissue and has also been designated as "infarct core." Areas of prolonged MTT, reduced CBF, but normal CBV are interpreted as (ischemic) penumbra. This combination of images suggests that compensatory mechanisms preserve CBV in what appears to be viable tissue.

Next is to determine the patient's eligibility for intravenous thrombolysis. Only intracranial hemorrhage, parenchymal intracranial malignancy, or a large established area of acute infarction represents clear imaging contraindications to IV tPA.[18] Imaging features, including volume of established infarction, presence and location of the clot, and degree of mismatch on perfusion imaging, all factor into patient selection for subsequent mechanical thrombectomy.

Patients with elevated blood pressure but otherwise eligible for treatment should have blood pressure reduced to ≤185/110 mmHg before administration of tPA. Care should be taken to reduce the blood pressure cautiously, particularly in the case of patients with a large-vessel syndrome, to avoid compromising collateral blood flow and then extending the area of ischemic brain.[1] Control of blood pressure continues after tPA administration, and targets after endovascular recanalization may be adjusted lower to avoid reperfusion injury.

The recommended dose of alteplase is 0.9 mg/kg, 10% given as a bolus and the remainder given as an infusion over 60 min (maximum dose 90 mg).[19] Once the decision is made to offer tPA to the patient, they must explain their recommendation clearly and thoroughly. Ideally, the patient should provide informed consent; however, when a patient cannot provide consent because of aphasia or anosognosia and a surrogate decision maker is not readily available, it is justified to proceed with treatment if there is a potentially severe disabling deficit.[1] The informed consent should include these basic elements: (1) nature of the decision,

(2) reasonable alternatives, (3) risks and benefits related to the proposed treatment and each alternative, and (4) assessment of patient understanding.

Patients eligible for mechanical thrombectomy should receive tPA if eligible and then proceed without delay to the angiography suite. Improvement with tPA alone may not be permanent, and many patients with a persistent occlusion may deteriorate. Criteria for endovascular clot retrieval include the following: (1) prestroke modified Rankin Scale score of 0–1, (2) occlusion of the internal carotid artery or middle cerebral artery (segment 1), (3) age ≥18 years, (4) NIHSS score ≥6, (5) Alberta Stroke Program Early CT Score of ≥6,[20] and (6) initiation of treatment within 6 h of symptom onset.[1] Additional selection criteria have been determined for patients presenting with large-vessel clinical syndromes >6 h from the onset of symptoms.[1]

THE PRESENTING CLINICAL PROBLEM

A 55-year-old man presents to the ED after falling on the floor at home. His spouse heard the thud and found him awake but struggling to get up with left-sided weakness and slightly slurred speech. On examination, the patient has an elevated blood pressure and a right hemispheric syndrome with anosognosia for his deficits. The learner must direct an "acute stroke code."

Learning objectives are shown in Table 5.1. To successfully complete the scenario, the learner should (1) take a focused history obtaining a clear time of onset or last-known normal time; (2) perform and score NIHSS, recognizing that the patient has a right hemispheric syndrome; (3) order and interpret a head CT scan and CT angiogram of the head and neck, identifying a right internal carotid artery occlusion; (4) lower the patient's blood pressure cautiously to <185/110 mmHg; (5) review the tPA checklist with the patient and his spouse and recommend treatment; (6) inform the patient and his spouse of the risks and benefits of treatment and obtain consent; (7) direct administration of tPA using the correct dose; and (8) activate the endovascular team for mechanical clot retrieval. Key competencies are summarized in Fig. 5.1.

Preparation

The patient lies on a hospital bed in the ED with a peripheral IV catheter inserted and vital signs showing on the monitor. Before the simulation, learners receive the 2018 guidelines for the management of acute ischemic stroke[1] to review in advance. Additional setup and equipment required are detailed in Table 5.2.

TABLE 5.1 Objectives
• Demonstrate a rapid, accurate assessment of a patient with acute ischemic stroke
• Perform NIHSS and score correctly
• Incorporate knowledge of inclusion/exclusion criteria for tPA into decision-making
• Identify hyperdense MCA on CT and carotid occlusion on CTA
• Identify anosognosia and consider in consent process
• Administer thrombolytics and proceed with endovascular retrieval of the clot

NIHSS, National Institutes of Health Stroke Scale; *tPA*, tissue-type plasminogen activator; *MCA*, middle cerebral artery; *CT*, computed tomography; *CTA*, CT angiogram.

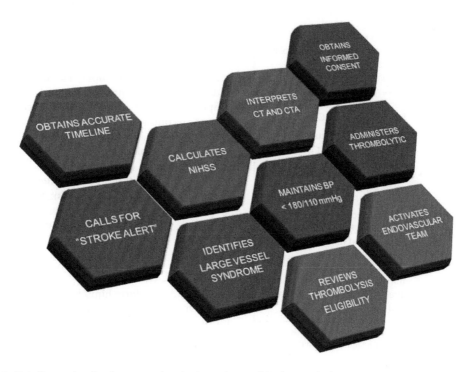

FIG. 5.1 Deconstructing key competencies in acute carotid artery occlusion.

Coaching Actors

Instructions to the actor are summarized in Table 5.3. Successful portrayal of a right hemispheric syndrome is challenging but, with clear instruction and practice, can be remarkably convincing. The actor should lie on the bed moving only the right arm and leg and looking only toward the right side of the room. If the learner stands on his left, the actor should look around the right side of the room as if trying to find the voice before answering the question. The actor should not seem confused and answers questions easily. Specifically the actor is oriented to person, place, date, and time and is able to report what happened correctly. However, the actor must convey that he feels normal and does not think that anything is currently wrong with him. Once these principles are established in the actor's mind, he or she can convincingly field any question from the learner.

It is helpful to tell the actor exactly what will happen. For example, "the learner may ask you to look straight ahead and count fingers in your peripheral vision. Keep looking towards the right side of the room. You

TABLE 5.2
Scenario Setup for Acute Carotid Artery Occlusion

People needed	• Actor to play the ED nurse • Actor to play the patient's spouse • Actor to play the patient • Attending physician or neurocritical care fellow to facilitate
Equipment needed	• 2 headsets (emergency nurse, facilitator) • Syringes and infusion bag • BP cuff • IV line • Oxygen by nasal cannula • Nicardipine, labetalol, alteplase, normal saline • Laboratory results • ECG with interpretation (atrial fibrillation) • NIH Stroke Scale Cards
Setup needed	• ED face sheet (include weight and height) in folder attached to the door • BP cuff on patient and IV line attached to the right antecubital fossa • Monitor showing atrial fibrillation, 190 BP/95 mmHg, normal heart rate and SpO2 in room air • Head CT on monitor (monitor turned off until learner requests imaging); CXR and CTA head and neck available

BP, blood pressure; *ED*, emergency department; *CXR*, chext x-ray; *IV*, intravenous catheter; *NIH*, National Institutes of Health; *SpO2*, peripheral capillary oxygen saturation.

can see the fingers on the right. You do not see fingers on the left side. If the learner moves directly in front of where you are looking, you still cannot see the fingers on your left side." The actor also must never move the left arm or leg and should allow them to fall heavily to the bed if the learner holds them up and lets go. The actor should report feeling on the right side of his face, arm, and leg but not the left. If the learner picks up his left arm to show him his left hand and asks whose hand it is, the actor should answer "yours." The actor should not try to simulate facial weakness or slurred speech.

The actor portraying the patient's spouse should receive a written history of present illness, past medical, social, and family history, as well as a review of systems and medication list. The most important information is highlighted for them to commit to memory (e.g., last-known normal time and absence of seizures, new incontinence, previous stroke, recent surgeries or procedures). When information is not provided in the script, the spouse should answer negatively. If the learner recommends thrombolysis without clearly explaining what it is as well as the risks and benefits, the spouse is instructed to ask those questions before providing consent ("are there risks?").

The nurse should provide realism and facilitate the flow of the scenario. The nurse may prompt the learner to examine the patient, direct them to neuroimaging if requested, and provide interventions at the learner's direction.

THE IDEAL LEARNER

L enters and introduces himself. He obtains a history of a fall 2 h ago without loss of consciousness or amnesia for the event, followed by onset of left-sided weakness and slurred speech. On hearing of the fall, he inquires about the presence of pain anywhere, which *P* denies.

TABLE 5.3
Instructions to Actors Before Simulation

• Completely ignore everything on the left side of the room (eyes and head looking to the right)

• Do not recognize your left hand as yours

• Mimic left-sided flaccidity

• Do not attempt to mimic slurred speech or facial paresis

• You do not recognize that your left side is weak (anosognosia)

• You can only see objects in the right side of your visual field (even with one eye closed)

• You cannot feel the left side of your face, arm, or leg

He reviews the patient's medications that include a statin and a β-blocker. While taking the patient's history, *L* observes a clear right gaze preference, left hemineglect, and left hemiplegia as well as a blood pressure of 190/95 mmHg. He instructs the nurse to give 10-mg IV labetalol and orders an urgent noncontrast head CT scan and CTA of the head and neck, chest X-ray, electrocardiogram, and laboratory tests including a complete blood count, basic chemistry panel, and international normalized ratio (INR) (INR 1.6). He then performs an NIHSS before *P* is taken to the CT scanner. *L* completes a rapid NIHSS assessment correctly and calculates a score of 15 for partial right gaze palsy, left homonymous hemianopia, hemiplegia, hemianesthesia, and hemineglect.

CONF shows *L* to the monitor, where he identifies a right hyperdense middle cerebral artery (MCA) sign (Fig. 5.2, left) and reports aloud that there is no hemorrhage or established infarction. He then reviews the CTA and reports an acute right carotid occlusion (Fig. 5.2, right). Looking to the monitor and, seeing that the BP is now 175/85 mmHg, he instructs CONF to mix the tPA. He tells *P*'s wife that he will ask a series of questions to determine whether it is safe to treat him with tPA. After excluding contraindications, *L* recommends treatment with tPA to *P*'s wife and informs her of the risks and benefits of treatment. He reports that the alternative is to not treat, in which case *P* may still improve but with a higher probability of permanent disability or death. *P*'s wife consents to tPA on

his behalf. *L* instructs CONF to give the tPA and states the correct dose and administration instructions. He instructs CONF to notify him if the BP is >185/110, and he activates the endovascular team. He then informs *P* and his wife about the carotid artery occlusion and recommends mechanical clot retrieval. Scenario ends.

THE NOT-SO-IDEAL LEARNER
We have identified the following common missteps:

1. *Learner does not clearly establish the time of symptom onset.* Some will assume that the onset was the time of the fall. Because it was unwitnessed and the patient has severe anosognosia for his deficits, that is unreliable. The time of onset should be the time he was last seen to be normal.

2. *Learner spends too much time on the history.* This tendency varies depending on the type of learner. Those used to practice in the emergency department are less prone to spend time on irrelevant historical information. In acute stroke care, valuable time (and neurons) can be lost by taking a too-detailed history.

3. *Learner delays administration of tPA unnecessarily.* The reasons may include waiting for INR or platelet count, failure to mix the tPA as soon as the decision to offer is made (waiting instead until the tPA checklist and consent are completed), or failure to lower blood pressure in anticipation of tPA treatment.

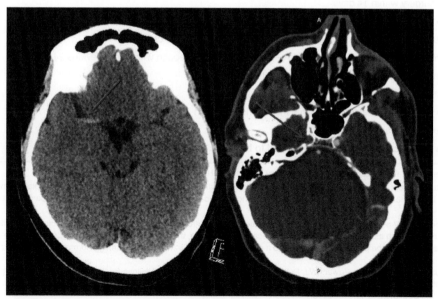

FIG. 5.2 Left: noncontrast head CT scan with right hyperdense middle cerebral artery sign (*arrow*); right: CT angiogram of the head shows filling defect due to clot in the right internal carotid artery (*arrow*).

4. *Learner does not order a CTA at the time of the CT scan.* This leads to a scenario where either mechanical clot retrieval is delayed while the patient is sent back to radiology for vascular imaging or the patient is sent to the endovascular suite without noninvasive vascular imaging. In the latter case, the interventionalist does not have information that may assist their approach (e.g., status of the collateral vessels, appearance of a dissection), and in some cases, there may be no large-vessel occlusion, which exposes the patient to the unnecessary risk of a cerebral angiography.

5. *The learner does not consider endovascular therapy.* Unfortunately, this denies the patient the opportunity to receive a now standard intervention.

ADAPTING THE SCENARIO

We have adapted this scenario in multiple ways. Novice neurology learners, emergency medicine residents, or critical care medicine fellows may be presented with a straightforward tPA case with no contraindications to allow them to practice taking a focused history, performing NIHSS, obtaining informed consent, and

---

TABLE 5.4
Checklist for tPA

INCLUSION CRITERIA
Age $\geq$18 years
Onset of symptoms within 3 h of "last-known normal time"
Onset of symptoms between 3 and 4.5 h of "last-known normal time" and NIHSS < 25

EXCLUSION CRITERIA
Head CT scan reveals an acute intracranial hemorrhage
Ischemic stroke within 3 months
Severe head trauma within 3 months
Intracranial/intraspinal surgery within 3 months
History of intracranial hemorrhage
Presenting symptoms and signs most consistent with subarachnoid hemorrhage
Major surgery within 14 days
Gastrointestinal malignancy or bleeding within 21 days
Coagulopathy: platelets < 100,000/mm^3, INR > 1.7, aPTT > 40 s, or PT > 15 s[a]
Patient received a treatment dose of low—molecular weight heparin within the previous 24 h
Thrombin inhibitors or direct thrombin inhibitors[b]
Patient is taking a glycoprotein IIb/IIIa receptor inhibitor
Acute ischemic stroke and symptoms most consistent with infective endocarditis
Intraaxial intracranial neoplasm
Acute ischemic stroke known or suspected to be associated with aortic arch dissection

INR, international normalized ratio; *NIHSS,* National Institutes of Health Stroke Scale.

[a] In patients without a history of coagulopathy and who are not taking anticoagulants, treatment with IV alteplase can be initiated before the availability of laboratory results but should be discontinued if results are not within the parameters listed here.

[b] Treatment with IV alteplase may be considered in patients taking direct thrombin inhibitors or direct factor Xa inhibitors if laboratory tests such as aPTT, INR, platelet count, ecarin clotting time, thrombin time, or appropriate direct factor Xa activity assays are normal or the patient has not received a dose of these agents for >48 h (assuming normal renal metabolizing function).

Table adapted from reference Powers WJ, Rabinstein AA, Ackerson T, et al. Guidelines for the early management of patients with acute ischemic stroke: a guideline for healthcare professionals from the American Heart Association/American Stroke Association. *Stroke.* 2018;49:e46—e110.

directing tPA administration with the proper dose and administration instructions. The scenario, as presented here, is designed for more advanced neurology residents as it is the knowledge required to direct tPA and endovascular therapy. We have also adapted this scenario in some instances to include having the patient develop a severe acute headache immediately after all have agreed to proceed with endovascular therapy. The learner must then manage the tPA-related intracranial hemorrhage (stop infusion and give IV tranexamic acid), reroute the patient to the ICU and consult a neurosurgeon after a CT scan. This adjustment of scenario is slightly contrived because acute hemorrhage during IV tPA infusion is uncommon, but it allows the learner to consider treatment options if this complication occurs.

DEBRIEFING

Debriefing is used to emphasize the key competencies. It could concentrate on a detailed discussion of the contraindications of IV thrombolysis (Table 5.4). The reasons for excluding patients can be discussed. The current completed clinical trials of endovascular treatment (and their patient selection criteria) can be briefly summarized and—if available—some additional challenging cases can be shown. The main purpose here is to reinforce to the learner the importance of efficiency and direct communication to expedite delivery of acute stroke therapies.

CONCLUSIONS

Acute stroke treatment has become a major intervention, and patients with an acute stroke are rarely admitted for rehabilitation alone. Competency and efficiency in the assessment and treatment of acute ischemic stroke require a significant knowledge of current clinical trials and their implications for treatment. Success in stroke care requires a methodical approach, strong communication, team leadership skills, and practice to deliver intravenous thrombolysis safely and organize endovascular retrieval as rapidly as possible in appropriate candidates.

REFERENCES

1. Powers WJ, Rabinstein AA, Ackerson T, et al. 2018 guidelines for the early management of patients with acute ischemic stroke: a guideline for healthcare professionals from the American Heart Association/American Stroke Association. *Stroke*. 2018;49:e46−e110.

2. Ibrahim F, Akhtar N, Salam A, et al. Stroke thrombolysis protocol shortens "door-to-needle time" and improves outcomes-experience at a tertiary care center in Qatar. *J Stroke Cerebrovasc Dis*. 2016;25:2043−2046.

3. McTaggart RA, Yaghi S, Cutting SM, et al. Association of a primary stroke center protocol for suspected stroke by large-vessel occlusion with efficiency of care and patient outcomes. *JAMA Neurol*. 2017;74:793−800.

4. Zuckerman SL, Magarik JA, Espaillat KB, et al. Implementation of an institution-wide acute stroke algorithm: improving stroke quality metrics. *Surg Neurol Int*. 2016;7: S1041−S1048.

5. Lansberg MG, Schrooten M, Bluhmki E, et al. Treatment time-specific number needed to treat estimates for tissue plasminogen activator therapy in acute stroke based on shifts over the entire range of the modified Rankin Scale. *Stroke*. 2009;40:2079−2084.

6. Lees KR, Bluhmki E, von Kummer R, et al. Time to treatment with intravenous alteplase and outcome in stroke: an updated pooled analysis of ECASS, ATLANTIS, NINDS, and EPITHET trials. *Lancet*. 2010;375:1695−1703.

7. Marler JR, Tilley BC, Lu M, et al. Early stroke treatment associated with better outcome: the NINDS rt-PA stroke study. *Neurology*. 2000;55:1649−1655.

8. Saver JL. Time is brain−quantified. *Stroke*. 2006;37: 263−266.

9. Nogueira RG, Jadhav AP, Haussen DC, et al. Thrombectomy 6 to 24 hours after stroke with a mismatch between deficit and infarct. *N Engl J Med*. 2018;378:11−21.

10. Saver JL, Goyal M, van der Lugt A, et al. Time to treatment with endovascular thrombectomy and outcomes from ischemic stroke: a meta-analysis. *JAMA*. 2016;316: 1279−1288.

11. Fonarow GC, Smith EE, Saver JL, et al. Improving door-to-needle times in acute ischemic stroke: the design and rationale for the American Heart Association/American Stroke Association's Target: stroke initiative. *Stroke*. 2011;42: 2983−2989.

12. Kamal N, Holodinsky JK, Stephenson C, et al. Improving door-to-needle times for acute ischemic stroke: effect of rapid patient registration, moving directly to computed tomography, and giving alteplase at the computed tomography scanner. *Circ Cardiovasc Qual Outcomes*. 2017;10.

13. Mehta T, Strauss S, Beland D, et al. Stroke simulation improves acute stroke management: a systems-based practice experience. *J Grad Med Educ*. 2018;10:57−62.

14. Tsivgoulis G, Katsanos AH, Schellinger PD, et al. Successful reperfusion with intravenous thrombolysis preceding mechanical thrombectomy in large-vessel occlusions. *Stroke*. 2018;49:232−235.

15. Prabhakaran S, Ruff I, Bernstein RA. Acute stroke intervention: a systematic review. *JAMA*. 2015;313:1451−1462.

16. Hacke W. A new DAWN for imaging-based selection in the treatment of acute stroke. *N Engl J Med*. 2018;378: 81−83.

17. Mistry EA, Mistry AM, Nakawah MO, et al. Mechanical thrombectomy outcomes with and without intravenous thrombolysis in stroke patients: a meta-analysis. *Stroke*. 2017;48:2450–2456.

18. Demaerschalk BM, Kleindorfer DO, Adeoye OM, et al. Scientific rationale for the inclusion and exclusion criteria for intravenous alteplase in acute ischemic stroke: a Statement for Healthcare Professionals from the American Heart Association/American Stroke Association. *Stroke*. 2016;47: 581–641.

19. National Institute of Neurological D, Stroke rt PASSG. Tissue plasminogen activator for acute ischemic stroke. *N Engl J Med*. 1995;333:1581–1587.

20. Barber PA, Demchuk AM, Zhang J, et al. Validity and reliability of a quantitative computed tomography score in predicting outcome of hyperacute stroke before thrombolytic therapy. ASPECTS Study Group. Alberta Stroke Programme Early CT Score. *Lancet*. 2000;355: 1670–1674.

CHAPTER 6

Simulating Basilar Artery Occlusion

The management of severe disabling stroke in the posterior circulation has changed and now requires a number of quick decisions. As discussed in Chapter 5, there are a multiplicity of clinical presentations and a large spectrum of neuroimaging findings that now need urgent evaluation. Clinicians in every specialty must juggle and accept (or discard) sets of data within minutes. Comprehensive stroke centers appropriately put the onus on achieving a fast intrahospital flow. For interventionalists, once access is achieved, the time to crossing the lesion and time to recanalization have become new metrics.

While time is critical in all acute stroke treatment, there may be more wiggle room with large-vessel posterior circulation stroke than in the anterior circulation. Endovascular experience in treatment of posterior circulation stroke is notably different with good recoveries even more than 24 h after onset. In this disorder, it is justifiable to open up the basilar artery no matter what, although exceptions to this rule exist (e.g., loss of most brainstem reflexes and already completed infarctions of all territories supplied by the basilar artery and its terminal branches).

Simulating acute disabling stroke—teaching urgent action with thrombolysis with or without endovascular thrombectomy—should include a comprehensive scenario on recognition and management of acute basilar artery occlusion for three reasons. First, embolus to the basilar artery may present with acute coma or a so-called "locked-in syndrome" (an awake state with minimal or no ability of the patient to respond to the examiner). These two cardinal neurologic conditions are part of the fundamentals of acute neurology and a requisite for each physician attending to these cases. Locked-in syndrome from an embolus in the basilar artery is such an iconic acute neurologic condition that it should be recognized in any emergency department and must, therefore, be practiced in the simulation center.[1–3] The abnormality is missed if the neurologic examination is truncated to a Glasgow Coma Scale (the FOUR Score which includes assessment of eye movements and brainstem reflexes will pick it up). Posterior circulation strokes are generally also not identified on the current NIH Stroke Scale

(NIHSS), which seriously complicates recognition in emergency departments, where neurologists are not the first responders and the NIHSS sometimes replaces a full neurologic examination.

Second, the disorder falls under the rubric of coma with "normal" CT (Chapter 8), which pertains to a relatively small number of disorders. The learner must mentally link a locked-in syndrome to the pons, anticipate a pontine lesion on CT but then, seeing nothing, reason that it must be early ischemia from an embolus to the basilar artery. Once the learner has diagnosed the disorder, the focus turns to the problem to the brainstem and, thus also, the posterior cerebral vasculature. Careful scrutiny of the CT scan will result in recognition of a key and often overlooked sign; namely, a hyperdense dot in the basilar artery.

Third, decisions regarding intervention are not time based (or time limited) as in anterior circulation stroke, and any acute worsening, despite fluctuating signs and symptoms days before, may be treatable with thrombolysis or, more commonly, endovascular retrieval of the clot.

In this chapter, we provide the building blocks to direct a scenario aimed at recognizing the more severely affected patient with a posterior circulation stroke. A detailed history from a proxy is often necessary if the patient presents unresponsive and intubated.

THE PROBLEM BEFORE US

Ischemic strokes in the posterior circulation account only for one in five of all ischemic strokes. Most strokes, are small and involve branch vessel occlusions. However, large-vessel (vertebral, basilar, and posterior cerebral artery) occlusions are less common. An acute embolus to the basilar artery is even more rarely seen by physicians, and therefore, the very low prevalence of this disorder hinders recognition. Ominous clinical signs include fluctuating (stuttering) weakness, clinical signs of rotational vertigo, diplopia, visual field cuts, and unsteady gait followed by unconsciousness or even an "out-of-the-blue," acute coma with motor posturing requiring emergent intubation. Although it should be possible—at least initially—in most cases of basilar artery occlusion to make a correct diagnosis,[4] clinical recognition of acute basilar artery occlusion is difficult for any physician because it requires a detailed, seldom-performed neurologic examination of the brainstem. Basilar artery embolization occurs mostly as a result of cardiogenic embolus, but a dissection of the vertebral artery can propagate easily into the wall of the basilar artery and close the lumen. A thrombus can also embolize to more distal parts of the basilar artery, including the tip, which may occlude both posterior cerebral arteries. When the embolus lodges in the mid-basilar area, it involves multiple penetrating arteries and may lead to significant pontine involvement, which may lead to a full or nearly complete locked-in syndrome. In any patient with major manifestations (e.g., oculomotor paresis, quadriparesis), emergent endovascular clot retrieval is necessary and, surprisingly, even in the most severe manifestations (such as locked-in syndrome), may lead to significant improvement.

Embolus to the basilar artery is usually acute, but ischemia may have occurred earlier. A thorough, well-taken history may reveal the presence of prior episodes of vertigo, nausea, and also a transient hemiparesis.[5] Involvement of the top of the basilar artery, where the superior cerebellar artery and posterior cerebral arteries branch off, may cause ischemia to the mesencephalon, thalami, inferior temporal lobes, and occipital lobes, which may cause signs and symptoms of acute diplopia, reduced gait, reduced or fluctuating consciousness, or moments of vigilance alternating with stupor. These patients develop a rostral brainstem infarction, a syndrome characterized by visual field defects, disorders of vertical gaze, convergence, a skew deviation, and pupillary abnormalities mostly resulting in small and poorly reactive pupils. Behavior abnormalities, including hallucinosis, are common. Visual field defects, including visual perseverations and scintillations in an optic field, have also been described. Many of the occipital infarcts are bilateral, and cortical blindness may be noted.

Patients with thalamic lesions cannot form new memories, and unfortunately, this may be permanent in patients with paramedian thalamic infarcts. In several other patients, a transient agitation and a frontal-like syndrome have been seen. Smaller brainstem infarcts have been described, and there are several brainstem syndromes with French and German eponyms (e.g., Weber, Foville, Millard−Gubler, Wallenberg) in which patients have a constellation of findings localized to specific, well-defined lesions in the pons, medulla, or even mesencephalon.

The most difficult-to-recognize patient is the one who appears comatose, requiring urgent intubation.[6,7] Recognition of a locked-in syndrome is very important, and every physician should be attentive to this possibility. As alluded to earlier, using the FOUR Score for initial coma examination will detect a locked-in syndrome.[8−11] Patients are basically deafferented, unresponsive (not the same as coma), and unable to communicate other than with vertical eye movements and blinking. This is one of the most devastating acute strokes, mostly because the patient's attempts at communication are not understood. Other important findings include the presence of anisocoria with a mid-position pupil on one side and a pinpoint pupil on the other, indicating interrupted reflex arches both in the mesencephalon and pons (Fig. 6.1).[12] Horizontal eye movements are absent.[13,14] The patient is mute from cerebellar involvement and, before intubation, may also have marked dysphagia and pooling secretions. Motor response, often in the more severe cases, is extensor posturing with an increased reflex pattern and bilateral Babinski signs. Many patients may present with "shivering" or "convulsions," which look like seizures to the uninitiated.[14] The key finding is to recognize locked-in syndrome and to find a hyperdense basilar artery sign on CT scan. Once this neurologic-radiologic link has been established, IV thrombolysis can be administered (within the 4½-h time window) followed by an urgent endovascular procedure to retrieve the clot. The current 4½-h time window from onset to administration of IV tPA can be determined by calculating when sudden worsening to a major deficit has occurred—mostly and justifiably ignoring the minor fluctuations so common in this disorder. This allows IV tPA administration in patients who could clearly benefit; in some, it may even result in complete resolution. Unfortunately, symptoms will return if the cerebral angiogram demonstrates a clot in the basilar artery that must be retrieved by endovascular means.

In any patient found unresponsive, the time course of onset is mostly unknown but not crucial in the treatment. The significant morbidity and mortality rates in patients with a mid-basilar artery occlusion warrant aggressive endovascular treatment to recanalize the basilar artery.

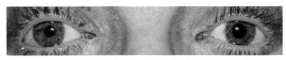

FIG. 6.1 Photo of pupil anisocoria (to be shown to learner).

THE PRESENTING CLINICAL PROBLEM

A 50-year-old male arrives in the emergency department (ED) after his wife found him unresponsive at home in the late evening. Apparently, he was normal before his wife left for work early in the morning, but the history also reveals prior vertigo attacks. His wife had noted intermittent stiffening and tremulousness of his extremities when she found him with a gurgling speech. When the paramedics arrived, they found him unresponsive but maintaining his own airway and ventilation. There was no evidence of trauma nor is there a prior history of seizures. The learners must discern whether the patient has an acute occlusion of the basilar artery and to recognize indications of locked-in syndrome.

The main objectives are to (1) differentiate locked-in syndrome from coma; (2) recognize that a comatose-appearing patient with a normal CT scan could have an infarct in the brainstem and/or bilateral thalami which is not visible on the CT scan; (3) recognize a hyperdense basilar artery on CT scan; and (4) acknowledge the urgency for thrombolytics and endovascular treatment. The key issues of the scenario are summarized in Fig. 6.2 and the objectives, in Table 6.1.

Preparation

The actor is placed on a hospital bed in the ED with a peripheral IV inserted and vital signs shown on a monitor. He has a blood pressure of 211/104 mmHg, normal heart rate, respiratory rate of 16, normal temperature, and adequate oxygenation. He is unresponsive and does not speak. The setup and equipment are detailed in Table 6.2.

Coaching the Actor

Actors will need clear, detailed coaching; the instructions are summarized in Table 6.3. In principle, the actor is instructed to be immobile and only move his eyes vertically with occasional blinking. There should be no verbal output if touched by the learner. The motor response should be forceful extension with both arms. The actor should receive instruction on extensor posturing and how to simulate triple-flexion response when the learner applies pressure to the nailbed of the toes. The breathing pattern is normal.

THE IDEAL LEARNER

L enters and, after introductions, obtains a history of prior episodic dizziness and resolved gait abnormalities. Most recently, the patient was found unresponsive in the afternoon (he last appeared normal 8 h previously). *CONF* also reveals that he witnessed an episode of shivering and posturing. It is important that *L* considers seizures, intoxication, hypoglycemia,

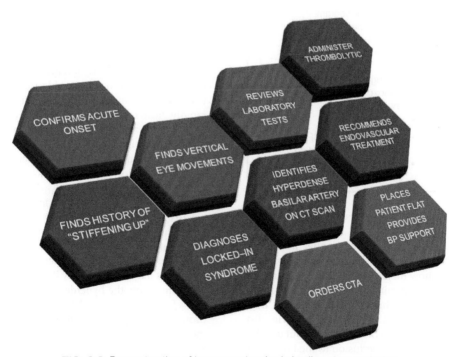

FIG. 6.2 Deconstruction of key competencies in basilar artery occlusion.

TABLE 6.1
Objectives

- Demonstrate the assessment of an unresponsive patient
- Obtain a focused assessment of the time of onset, pertinent past medical history and laboratory evaluation
- Recognize locked-in syndrome
- Identify hyperdense basilar artery on CT
- Incorporate knowledge of eligibility criteria for tPA into decision-making
- Recognize indications for endovascular intervention in basilar artery occlusion

TABLE 6.2
Simulation Scenario Setup for Basilar Artery Occlusion

People needed	<ul><li>Actor to play ED nurse</li><li>Patient (actor)</li><li>Attending physician or neurocritical care fellow to facilitate</li></ul>
Equipment needed	<ul><li>ED face sheet with summary of the history</li><li>Electrocardiogram</li><li>Actual imaging results of a real patient—brain CT, CTA</li><li>Laboratory results</li><li>tPA</li><li>Syringes</li><li>Naloxone syringe (0.04 mg)</li><li>IV line</li><li>BP cuff</li></ul>
Setup needed	<ul><li>Monitor showing BP 211/104 mmHg, atrial fibrillation, HR 96</li><li>Patient lying in bed (head of bed at 30 degrees)</li></ul>

and stroke. *L* excludes hypoglycemia after laboratory studies show normal glucose. The laboratory studies provided to him show no abnormalities of any concern including a normal troponin. He recognizes the patient has a slightly depressed breathing frequency. *L* may consider naloxone to treat opioid overdose. He also notes a minor increase in *P*'s blood pressure but decides not to treat it, knowing that perfusion to the brainstem must be guaranteed. Instead, he lays the patient flat and

requests a 1-L bolus of normal saline considering that the patient was found down. *L* examines the patient and finds only vertical eye movements and blinking and subsequently determines that *P* is in a locked-in state. He then reviews the CT scan (Fig. 6.3) and identifies a hyperdense basilar sign and no evidence of ischemic stroke in the cerebellum or pons. *L* associates clinical findings with the hyperdense basilar artery sign as an ischemia in the brainstem. *CONF* asks what is happening to the patient. If *L* recognizes basilar artery occlusion, he must consider whether the patient is eligible for IV tPA. If *L* does not mention tPA, *CONF* can ask "What about tPA?" *L* should then state that tPA cannot be administered without knowing the time of onset. *CONF* will ask if anything can be done for the patient ("Is it too late for any treatment?"). *L* should inform him that endovascular clot retrieval could be attempted after the cerebral angiogram confirms a clot in the basilar artery and that this is the only way to definitive improvement. *CONF* will ask if a transport cart is needed to take the patient to the angiogram suite, whereupon *L* requests transport to the angiography suite, and the scenario ends.

THE NOT-SO-IDEAL LEARNER

1. *L does not recognize locked-in syndrome.* *L* considers the patient "unresponsive" with little further specification. Moreover, *L* considers the adventitious movements to represent seizures and does not recognize that convulsions and extensor posturing might be consistent with a basilar artery occlusion.
2. *L sticks with the diagnosis of coma.* Several learners in our training have not been able to distinguish between a locked-in syndrome and coma and become rapidly flustered if the CT scan is interpreted as normal. (See also Chapter 8 on simulation of coma with a normal CT scan.) This often ends the scenario, as no further action is undertaken and no resolution follows. This leads to a thorough debriefing.
3. *L recognizes stroke in the basilar artery clinically but does not recognize a clot in the basilar artery on CT scan.* Often, however, learners pursue a CTA or a cerebral angiogram, which leads to the correct diagnosis. The error of not recognizing a hyperdense basilar artery sign is not major, particularly if the learner considers it but discounts the hyperdensity as insignificant.
4. *L asks for labetalol to treat hypertension.* This leads to a drop in blood pressure and loss of vertical movement, which suggests an ischemic pons. This will end the scenario unless the learner pursues a CTA and, subsequently, the correct treatment.

TABLE 6.3
Actor Instructions Before Simulation

- Lie with eyes closed.
- Demonstrate difficulty opening eyes and keeping them open but able to open both slowly.
- Breathe approximately 8–10 times per minute.
- Learner may hold your eyelids open to help and should allow you to blink occasionally.
- If learner asks you to look to the right or left or follow his finger laterally, do not move your eyes. If asked to look up or down, you can do it reliably.
- If the learner asks you to "look up for yes; look down for no" and then asks questions, you can respond in this manner.
- Try not to move your face too much; however, blinking is okay.
- Do not speak.
- If asked to cough, do not make any effort to do so. You can swallow if needed, but try to be as motionless as possible.
- If asked to move arms or legs up, make no effort to do so.
- If the learner holds your arms or legs up off the bed, allow them to fall limply to the bed when released.
- If the learner states he/she is applying pain (e.g., sternal rub, nasal pressure), extend your arms and legs as demonstrated.
- If the learner touches the bottom of your foot, bend your knee, pull your foot up, and raise your big toe (triple flexion) as demonstrated.

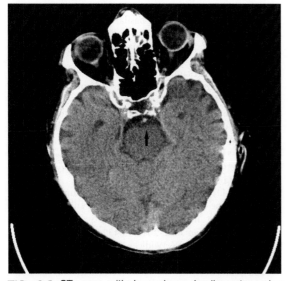

FIG. 6.3 CT scan with hyperdense basilar artery sign (arrow).

"Permissive hypertension" is a necessity in this disorder, and patients can improve with a marginally better blood pressure.

5. *L does not consider endovascular treatment as an option.* There is a general consensus among strokeologists that acute occlusions of the posterior circulation can be retrieved with a much longer time window—even up to 24 h.

ADAPTING THE SCENARIO

This scenario is difficult for any physician and, therefore, can be adapted and better facilitated with *CONF* providing more cues; for example, telling *L* that the patient is constantly blinking and questioning if the patient might be aware. In addition, *CONF* can remind *L* of the prior symptoms of vertigo and gait abnormality, which also suggest posterior circulation transient ischemic attacks.

DEBRIEFING

Debriefing in this scenario has several important components. First is the recognition of an important neurologic emergency when an embolus to the mid-basilar artery produces a locked-in syndrome. Depending on the learner, a brief synopsis of neurologic findings can be discussed (Table 6.4). The debriefing can include a discussion of the mechanisms of a locked-in syndrome, and it should be emphasized that the patient is able to hear as well as feel pain. The discussion can then proceed with neuroimaging of basilar artery occlusion and the absence of CT scan abnormalities when patients are seen shortly after onset. Second, the debriefing can also touch on the flaws of ordering an MRI scan, which would delay treatment. A more extensive discussion can follow on the benefits of endovascular clot retrieval, the absence of a clear timeline, the potential for significant

TABLE 6.4
Cardinal Symptoms of Basilar Artery Occlusion and Involved Brain Structures[2]

Symptoms	Brain Structure
Reduced consciousness or coma	Ascending reticular activating system
Reduced or irregular breathing patterns (apnea)	Nuclei of the pons and medulla oblongata
Dysarthria and bulbar symptoms	Cerebellum and cranial nerve nuclei of the medulla oblongata
Ophthalmoplegia, double vision, nystagmus	Cerebellum and the oculomotor nuclei of the brainstem
Ptosis, anisocoria	Mesencephalon, thalamus
Dysequilibrium, falling	Cerebellum and the brainstem cranial nerve nuclei regulating balance
Blindness, visual field deficits	Occipital lobes
Ataxia, loss of coordination of limbs and body	Cerebellum and linked proprioception and motor tracts
Bilateral motor and sensory paresis	Pontine pyramidal tracts, tegmentum, spinothalamic tract
Extension, rigidity, and shivering	Pontine pyramidal tracts

Adapted from Lindsberg PJ, Sairanen T, Strbian D, et al. Current treatment of basilar artery occlusion. *Ann N Y Acad Sci.* 2012;1268: 35–44.

recovery after clot retrieval, and general outcome of basilar artery occlusion.

The debriefing should devote some time to the potential early benefits of permissive hypertension, maintaining euvolemia, and actions such as placing the body flat or in Trendelenburg. The contraindication of IV thrombolysis (often outside the usual 4½-h time interval) requires discussion.

CONCLUSION

Acute basilar artery occlusion producing a locked-in syndrome offers the opportunity to teach a classic neurologic finding as well as a classic neurologic

disorder. When they present in combination, they are difficult to recognize, generally rarely seen, and usually missed or belatedly recognized. Once detected, there are major immediate therapeutic implications, and virtually all patients are transported to the neuroendovascular suite for microcatheter aspiration or retrieval of the clot.[15]

REFERENCES

1. Lindsberg PJ, Pekkola J, Strbian D, et al. Time window for recanalization in basilar artery occlusion: speculative synthesis. *Neurology.* 2015;85:1806–1815.
2. Lindsberg PJ, Sairanen T, Strbian D, et al. Current treatment of basilar artery occlusion. *Ann N Y Acad Sci.* 2012; 1268:35–44.
3. Schonewille WJ, Wijman CA, Michel P, et al. Treatment and outcomes of acute basilar artery occlusion in the Basilar Artery International Cooperation Study (BASICS): a prospective registry study. *Lancet Neurol.* 2009;8: 724–730.
4. Braksick SA, Wijdicks EFM. An NIHSS of 0 and a very disabling stroke. *Neurocrit Care.* 2017;26:444–445.
5. Mattle HP, Arnold M, Lindsberg PJ, et al. Basilar artery occlusion. *Lancet Neurol.* 2011;10:1002–1014.
6. Caplan LR. "Top of the basilar" syndrome. *Neurology.* 1980;30:72–79.
7. Demel SL, Broderick JP. Basilar occlusion syndromes: an update. *Neurohospitalist.* 2015;5:142–150.
8. Iyer VN, Mandrekar JN, Danielson RD, et al. Validity of the FOUR score coma scale in the medical intensive care unit. *Mayo Clin Proc.* 2009;84:694–701.
9. Stead LG, Wijdicks EF, Bhagra A, et al. Validation of a new coma scale, the FOUR score, in the emergency department. *Neurocrit Care.* 2009;10:50–54.
10. Wijdicks EF, Bamlet WR, Maramattom BV, et al. Validation of a new coma scale: the FOUR score. *Ann Neurol.* 2005;58: 585–593.
11. Wijdicks EF, Kramer AA, Rohs Jr T, et al. Comparison of the Full Outline of UnResponsiveness score and the Glasgow Coma Scale in predicting mortality in critically ill patients. *Crit Care Med.* 2015;43:439–444.
12. Burns JD, Schiefer TK, Wijdicks EF. Large and small: a tell-tale sign of acute pontomesencephalic injury. *Neurology.* 2009;72:1707.
13. Moncayo J, Bogousslavsky J. Vertebro-basilar syndromes causing oculo-motor disorders. *Curr Opin Neurol.* 2003; 16:45–50.
14. Ropper AH. 'Convulsions' in basilar artery occlusion. *Neurology.* 1988;38:1500.
15. Chiang CC, Dumitrascu OM, Wingerchuk DM, O'Carroll CB. Acute basilar artery occlusion: does recanalization improve clinical outcome? A critically appraised topic. *Neurologist.* 2018;23:71–74.

CHAPTER 7

Simulating Aneurysmal Subarachnoid Hemorrhage

Aneurysmal subarachnoid hemorrhage (SAH) is a neurologic and neurosurgical emergency that demands multidisciplinary expertise to recognize and rapidly treat the neurologic and (numerous) systemic complications. Many patients present with isolated severe headache but normal neurologic examination and appear solidly stable, but such an interpretation can result in a false sense of security. Early new manifestations include acute significant worsening and coma from rerupture hours after admission or gradually becoming more drowsy from obstructive hydrocephalus. Approximately 5%–10% of patients will experience rebleeding in the first 24 h.[1] Because rebleeding is associated with acute coma from a surge in intracranial pressure (ICP) and thus, higher mortality and increased morbidity among survivors, early aneurysm repair should be undertaken when possible.[1–3] Rebleeding may also present with a new seizure or new extensor posturing.[4,5] Acute hydrocephalus, as a result of blood-plugging arachnoid granulations or cisterns necessary for adequate cerebrospinal fluid circulation, occurs in approximately 20%–30% of patients, typically becoming symptomatic within the first 24–48 h but often rapidly improving with cerebrospinal fluid diversion.[6–8]

Recognizing the archetypal features of the headache that characterize aneurysmal rupture—the so-called "thunderclap headache"[2]—as well as the clinical presentation of both aneurysmal rebleeding and symptomatic hydrocephalus requires expert knowledge and experience. Because the consequences are so great and many specialties can become involved, we think a simulation scenario on SAH can be instructive. This simulation scenario will focus on the clinical recognition of SAH, rebleeding, obstructive hydrocephalus, and their management. Chapter 8 will focus on management of another common and serious complication—delayed cerebral ischemia from cerebral vasospasm.

THE PROBLEM BEFORE US

The clinical presentation of SAH is distinctive. Patients either suddenly become unresponsive without recovery of consciousness, or they describe an extremely sudden, unexpectedly severe headache with many vomiting acutely. The headache may be associated with brief loss of consciousness or focal neurologic deficits. It should be noted that one in 10 patients die before reaching the hospital or become brain dead soon after admission.[2]

Some patients report a less severe headache weeks preceding the SAH, and the occurrence of this warning—or sentinel—headache, because it indicates an unstable aneurysmal dome, increases the odds of rebleeding 10-fold.[9] When SAH is suspected, diagnosis is confirmed by CT scan, which has nearly perfect sensitivity for detecting subarachnoid blood when it is obtained within hours of the onset of this characteristic headache.[2,10]

The clinical course in poor-grade aneurysmal SAH is unpredictable in the first 24–48 h. Comatose patients with intact brainstem reflexes at presentation may improve in a matter of hours even without much neurosurgical or medical intervention. Serious early complications of SAH include rebleeding and hydrocephalus. Rebleeding typically occurs very early, within the first 12–24 h, and results in increased rates of mortality and poor functional outcomes. The common clinical features of rebleeding are coma associated with loss of several brainstem reflexes including pupillary light response and oculocephalic responses. In most patients, respiratory arrest or gasping breathing occurs, necessitating immediate endotracheal intubation and mechanical ventilation. Early identification and treatment of the aneurysm is thus recommended to reduce the rate of rebleeding.[2] Blood pressure should be controlled with a rapid-onset, titratable drug to balance the risk of increased aneurysmal - wall stress and maintenance of cerebral perfusion pressure before aneurysmal repair.[2] Specific blood pressure parameters have not been strictly defined, but empirically, a systolic blood pressure of <160 mm Hg is recommended pending further study.[2,11] Treating with an antifibrinolytic agent such as tranexamic acid or aminocaproic acid may reduce the risk of rebleeding until the aneurysm can be secured. These drugs are not continued for more than 72 h.

The other major early complication of aneurysmal SAH is obstructive hydrocephalus, which is frequently associated with rebleeding as a result of a ventricular clot blocking apertures and foramina but which may also occur after a first rupture. Acute hydrocephalus causes a—mostly insidious—decline in consciousness, eyes pointing downward, small pupils, and bradycardia. Cerebrospinal fluid diversion via ventricular or lumbar drainage, depending on the severity of clinical findings, is required and often leads to rapid improvement in responsiveness, ophthalmoparesis, and pupil size.

Patients who present with coma or who experience rebleeding after initially presenting as a good clinical grade may have diffuse cerebral edema. These patients often require intubation, a controlled mode of ventilation, and elevation of the head of the bed to 30 degrees to facilitate venous drainage. They may additionally benefit from hyperosmolar therapy and transient hyperventilation.

There are a number of immediate systemic complications in poor-grade SAH with cardiogenic shock from stress cardiomyopathy or myocardial injury, cardiac arrhythmias, and neurogenic pulmonary edema. Because aneurysmal SAH may present with several different clinical syndromes, a number of simulation scenarios can be built with increasing complexity.

THE PRESENTING CLINICAL PROBLEM

A 51-year-old woman presents to the ED for evaluation of a "worst-ever," split-second headache that developed when she lifted a heavy box. To discern whether learners recognize and can manage the early complications of aneurysmal SAH, the patient should describe her symptoms when asked. After the learner elicits a history of thunderclap headache and orders a CT scan, the patient has a brief convulsion and an acute increase in blood pressure followed by unresponsiveness. The scan can show diffuse subarachnoid blood and hydrocephalus.

The main objectives of this scenario are to (1) elicit a history of thunderclap headache, (2) diagnose aneurysmal rebleeding, (3) recognize and treat acutely increased intracranial pressure, (4) appreciate symptomatic hydrocephalus after rebleeding, and (5) request emergent neurosurgical evaluation for ventriculostomy placement (Table 7.1). Key issues of the scenario are summarized in Fig. 7.1.

Preparation

The mannequin is placed in a hospital bed in the ED with a peripheral intravenous catheter inserted and vital signs showing on the monitor. Two weeks before the simulation, learners receive aneurysmal SAH guidelines [2,3] to review in advance of the scenario. Additional setup and equipment required are detailed in Table 7.2.

Coaching Actors

The instructor can choose to use actors or mannequins for this scenario (instructions for coaching live actors are shown in Table 7.3). However, we typically prefer using a mannequin as the simulated patient (*P*) to simulate changes after the rebleeding event. The mannequin allows for closure of eyes, off-blink setting, fixed

---

TABLE 7.1 Objectives
• Recognize thunderclap headache
• Request neuroimaging after acute neurologic deterioration
• Find pupil change and recognize Cushing reflex
• Interpret neuroimaging correctly, recognizing both subarachnoid hemorrhage and hydrocephalus
• Request intubation and brief hyperventilation
• Treat initial acute hypertension
• Administer hyperosmolar therapy
• Administer an antifibrinolytic agent
• Request emergent neurosurgical evaluation for ventriculostomy placement and aneurysm treatment

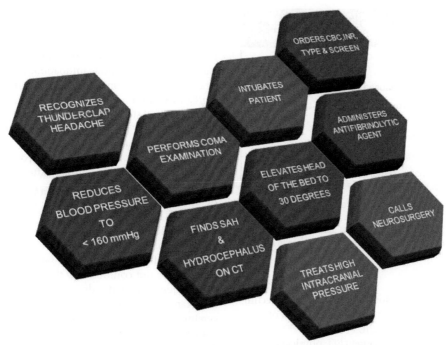

FIG. 7.1 Deconstructing key competencies in aneurysmal subarachnoid hemorrhage.

TABLE 7.2 **Scenario Setup for Aneurysmal Subarachnoid Hemorrhage**	
People needed	• SimMan 3G • Simulation technician to control the monitor • Actor to play the emergency medicine physician • Attending physician or neurocritical care fellow to facilitate
Equipment needed	• Two headsets (emergency physician, facilitator) • Syringes • BP cuff • IV line • Oxygen by nasal cannula • Mannitol, tranexamic acid, labetalol, normal saline • Intubation tray • Laboratory results
Setup needed	• Monitor showing sinus rhythm, elevated BP, normal heart rate, normal respiratory rate and SpO$_2$ on room air • Head CT on monitor (monitor turned off until learner requests imaging) • SimMan 3G on hospital bed (BP cuff, ECG leads, pulse oximetry, peripheral IV ×2 attached)

BP, blood pressure; *IV*, intravenous catheter; *SpO$_2$*, peripheral capillary oxygen saturation.

and dilated pupils, and "convulsions." The facilitator serves as the voice of the mannequin, answering the learner's questions without using the term "thunderclap headache." The facilitator should remember to use colloquial phrases such as "it hurt so bad, I had to sit down," "felt like I was going to vomit," "thought I might pass out," "came on from one second to the next," and avoid saying "worst headache of my life" but, if asked by the learner, answers "yes." The facilitator also initiates a brief convulsion and stops responding to

---

TABLE 7.3
Technician/Actor Instructions Before Simulation

- Describe key characteristics of a thunderclap headache.
- Describe feelings of nausea.
- Describe sudden worsening headache and then become unresponsive.
- Display labored breathing.[a]
- Display brief jitters in extremities.[a]
- Once unresponsive, remain so with eyes closed for remainder of scenario.[a]
- Do not respond to voice or nailbed pressure. You may act out extensor posturing.[a]

[a] Additional instructions for use when an actor is chosen in lieu of a mannequin.

---

the learner. It is at this point that the simulation technician changes the mannequin's settings such that one pupil is dilated and fixed to light.

The role of the confederate (ED physician) is to provide a natural flow to the scenario. The ED physician may ask what the learner thinks is going on and if there is anything that she should get started. Following the patient's loss of consciousness, she may prompt the learner to examine the patient, direct the learner to neuroimaging if requested, and provide interventions at the learner's direction. Intubation may be needed when indicated.

THE IDEAL LEARNER

L enters and introduces himself to P and $CONF$ after review of the ED face sheet. On hearing P's description of a severe, sudden-onset headache after lifting a heavy box, L thinks "thunderclap headache" and asks "how long did it take for the pain to get to maximal intensity? Was it seconds, minutes, or hours?" P reports that it was not there one second and was there the next. She mentions that she had to sit down on the floor because of the pain.

L notes the blood pressure of 190/120 mm Hg on the monitor and asks $CONF$ to give 10 mg intravenous labetalol. L then requests an urgent head CT scan, electrocardiogram, and laboratory studies including a complete blood count, chemistry, coagulation panel, type and screen, and troponin. Before the results come back, P suddenly develops a severe headache, has a series of convulsions, and becomes unresponsive. Blood pressure increases to 210/155 mm Hg. Heart rate decreases to 60 beats/min. When $CONF$ suggests

administration of lorazepam, L examines P and notes a lack of eye opening to pain and a unilateral fixed and dilated pupil. Suspecting aneurysmal SAH with rerupture and increased intracranial pressure with Cushing reflex, L requests intubation, hyperventilation, head-of-bed elevation to 30 degrees, administration of 1 g/kg of mannitol, and again asks about the head CT scan and requested labs. Anticipating a blood pressure drop with these measures, L prioritizes them over an additional dose of labetalol.

$CONF$ provides L with the requested studies and intubates P while L reviews them. After intubation, the ventilator rate is set to 30 breaths/min, and the head of the bed is elevated. While $CONF$ administers mannitol, L describes the head CT, noting aloud presence of diffuse SAH, filling of cisterns and fissures, and marked enlargement of ventricles reflecting acute hydrocephalus (Fig. 7.2). The laboratory results are normal and not confounding the examination.

L requests urgent administration of intravenous tranexamic acid and, appreciating a need for emergent cerebrospinal fluid diversion, requests an emergent neurosurgical consultation for ventriculostomy placement and treatment of the aneurysm. Observing a blood pressure of 180/92 mm Hg and heart rate of 50 bpm, L recommends initiation of a nicardipine infusion with instructions to maintain the systolic blood pressure <160 mm Hg. L then re-examines P, noting normalization of the pupils but no change in level of consciousness, and indicates CSF diversion with a ventriculostomy is urgent. The scenario ends.

THE NOT-SO-IDEAL LEARNER

We have identified the following common missteps:

1. *Ineffective history-taking skills*: Learner does not elicit a history of thunderclap headache. Because this is crucial for further flow of the scenario, $CONF$ can provide a history of acutely severe headache, a headache never experienced before. This should lead to review of the CT scan.

2. *Posturing is mistaken for a seizure*: Learner starts treatment with lorazepam and other antiseizure drugs, delaying further evaluation and critically delaying CSF diversion for treatment of life-threatening hydrocephalus. Debriefing should discuss how extensor posturing with a surge in ICP can mimic a seizure.

3. *Acute hypertension is not appreciated or not treated*: This may—theoretically—increase the risk of rebleeding again, but on the other hand, treatment is problematic if there is a Cushing reflex due to acutely increased intracranial pressure. Using beta blockade

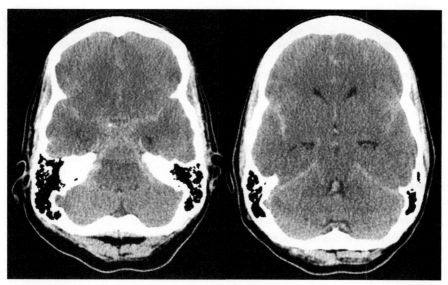

FIG. 7.2 Head CT scan showing aneurysmal subarachnoid hemorrhage with acute hydrocephalus.

may be contraindicated if there is bradycardia as it can precipitate a serious bradyarrhythmia.

4. *Learner does not examine the patient after she becomes unresponsive and misses the fixed dilated pupil*: This results in lack of recognition of brain compression and a lost opportunity to treat with hyperventilation and hyperosmolar therapy.

5. *Learner does not recognize hydrocephalus*: This is all too common and a justification for the simulation scenario. This delays treatment, which may result in worsening neurologic injury and, if left untreated long enough, a fatal bradyarrhythmia.

ADAPTING THE SCENARIO

This scenario can be easily adapted in several ways. For novice learners, the scenario can focus on the clinical history and initial management of SAH by presenting a good-grade SAH without the acute deterioration. The scenario can be made more challenging for advanced neurology, neurosurgery, emergency medicine, or anesthesiology learners (as rebleeding can be encountered during coiling or clipping) by simulating a Cushing reflex before proper intervention.

Poor-grade patients may present with acutely severe pulmonary edema and stress cardiomyopathy. Stress cardiomyopathy is fairly common with poor-grade SAH, and it can be observed clinically and on repeat echocardiograms. Images of poor ventricular function and regional-wall motion abnormalities with immobility of the apex can be shown on an echocardiogram image (or recording). Another opportunity exists to teach the management of acute cardiac arrhythmia with a significant decrease in blood pressure. Life-threatening cardiac arrhythmias are brief ventricular tachycardia, asystole, and torsades de pointes. Moreover, the scenario could focus on management of neurogenic pulmonary edema, which presents with marked hypoxemic respiratory failure (hypoxemia, greatly increased A–a gradient). Management of neurogenic pulmonary edema focuses on recruitment of collapsed alveoli with positive end-expiratory pressure (PEEP) to correct the marked ventilation-perfusion mismatch. PEEP alone should be sufficient to resolve neurogenic pulmonary edema, and weaning can be achieved rapidly in many patients when the acute catecholemine surge has subsided. If the origin of pulmonary edema is unclear or possibly confounded by cardiac injury, inotropes to improve ventricular forward flow could be considered.[12] These additional complexities can be added for general critical care or neurocritical care fellows.

DEBRIEFING

The debriefing is used to discuss the experience of managing this major neurologic emergeny. For some, it may

TABLE 7.4
Major Clinical Characteristics of Aneurysmal Subarachnoid Hemorrhage

- Split-second, never-before-experienced, severe headache
- Vomiting often with worsening headache
- Persistent, excruciating, poorly responsive to medication
- Focal signs rare (aphasia, hemiparesis, ophthalmoparesis)
- Presenting alert; coma or stupor is less common
- Nuchal rigidity is uncommon early but appears later
- Gradual decline indicates worsening hydrocephalus
- Acute decline indicates rebleeding
- Seizures may be present in stuporous patients
- CT scan is diagnostic in over 90% of cases
- CSF is diagnostic in less than 1% of cases with negative scan
- Other causes may exist in 10% of cases

be the first high-acuity situation they independently manage. The main characteristics of the first hour of aneurysmal SAH are shown in Table 7.4. This scenario highlights two serious, early complications of SAH: rebleeding and hydrocephalus. We emphasize the following three main teaching points: (1) the importance of early aggressive blood pressure control and administration of an antifibrinolytic to reduce the risk of rebleeding, (2) recognition and emergent management of increased intracranial pressure, and (3) recognition of hydrocephalus and the need for emergent ventriculostomy.

CONCLUSIONS

Learners have an opportunity to diagnose SAH and then independently direct its management. It is a unique situation in which the learner gets to think through and triage the order of interventions during a typical neurologic emergency in which multiple interventions are required. Management of SAH—as has often been said—is critical in the first (golden) hour of presentation.[12–14] Not only is its correct recognition important (made easy with a CT scan), but early interventions to treat or prevent complications improve the patient's chance at achieving a good outcome. This includes the administration of antifibrinolytics, placement of a ventriculostomy, and rapid treatment of the ruptured aneurysm once demonstrated by cerebral angiogram.

REFERENCES

1. Fujii Y, Takeuchi S, Sasaki O, et al. Ultra-early rebleeding in spontaneous subarachnoid hemorrhage. *J Neurosurg.* 1996;84:35–42.
2. Connolly Jr ES, Rabinstein AA, Carhuapoma JR, et al. Guidelines for the management of aneurysmal subarachnoid hemorrhage: a guideline for healthcare professionals from the American Heart Association/American Stroke Association. *Stroke.* 2012;43:1711–1737.
3. Diringer MN, Bleck TP, Claude Hemphill 3rd J, et al. Critical care management of patients following aneurysmal subarachnoid hemorrhage: recommendations from the Neurocritical Care Society's Multidisciplinary Consensus Conference. *Neurocrit Care.* 2011;15:211–240.
4. Claassen J, Peery S, Kreiter KT, et al. Predictors and clinical impact of epilepsy after subarachnoid hemorrhage. *Neurology.* 2003;60:208–214.
5. Molyneux AJ, Kerr RS, Yu LM, et al. International subarachnoid aneurysm trial (ISAT) of neurosurgical clipping versus endovascular coiling in 2143 patients with ruptured intracranial aneurysms: a randomized comparison of effects on survival, dependency, seizures, rebleeding, subgroups, and aneurysm occlusion. *Lancet.* 2005;366:809–817.
6. Hasan D, Vermeulen M, Wijdicks EF, et al. Management problems in acute hydrocephalus after subarachnoid hemorrhage. *Stroke.* 1989;20:747–753.
7. Heros RC. Acute hydrocephalus after subarachnoid hemorrhage. *Stroke.* 1989;20:715–717.
8. van Gijn J, Hijdra A, Wijdicks EF, et al. Acute hydrocephalus after aneurysmal subarachnoid hemorrhage. *J Neurosurg.* 1985;63:355–362.
9. Brisman JL, Song JK, Newell DW. Cerebral aneurysms. *N Engl J Med.* 2006;355:928–939.

10. Perry JJ, Stiell IG, Sivilotti ML, et al. Sensitivity of computed tomography performed within six hours of onset of headache for diagnosis of subarachnoid haemorrhage: prospective cohort study. *BMJ*. 2011;343:d4277.

11. Ohkuma H, Tsurutani H, Suzuki S. Incidence and significance of early aneurysmal rebleeding before neurosurgical or neurological management. *Stroke*. 2001;32: 1176–1180.

12. Rabinstein AA, Lanzino G. Aneurysmal subarachnoid hemorrhage: unanswered questions. *Neurosurg Clin N Am*. 2018;29:255–262.

13. Long B, Koyfman A, Runyon MS. Subarachnoid hemorrhage: updates in diagnosis and management. *Emerg Med Clin North Am*. 2017;35:803–824.

14. Lawton MT, Vates GE. Subarachnoid hemorrhage. *N Engl J Med*. 2017;377:257–266.

CHAPTER 8

Simulating Delayed Cerebral Ischemia

Most neurointensivists anticipate worsening after aneurysmal subarachnoid hemorrhage (SAH), cerebral vasospasm is the most difficult complication to manage. Obviously, the severity of neurological impairment on presentation is one of the strongest predictors of outcome after aneurysmal SAH. Patients who present alert with no localizing findings or who improve rapidly after cerebral resuscitation may experience excellent functional outcomes with careful management.[1] However, some will improve only to deteriorate after appearing misleadingly stable for days in the unit.

Delayed neurological deterioration is common following aneurysmal SAH and encompasses any objective decline in neurologic function that occurs after initial stabilization with the exception of rebleeding.[2,3] Patients may experience acute hydrocephalus, diffuse early cerebral edema, diffuse or focal cerebral ischemia, seizures, central fever, and disorders of sodium homeostasis, all of which can contribute to a change in neurologic status.

Cerebral vasospasm is the arterial narrowing after SAH that can lead to reduced cerebral blood flow and oxygen delivery, but many patients with vasospasm are asymptomatic, or they later may develop cerebral ischemia resulting in infarction. Delayed cerebral ischemia (DCI), defined as any neurologic deterioration thought to result from ischemia, should be considered if it lasts at least 1 h without another known cause.[3] The pathophysiology is likely far more complex, involving microthrombosis, cortical spreading depolarizations, and a number of biochemical derangements and neuroinflammation, but none of these mechanisms have yet led to effective targeted therapies.[4]

In general, early complications (within 24 h) after SAH include rebleeding and acute hydrocephalus (within 48 h), while cerebral vasospasm characteristically starts between 3 and 5 days after aneurysmal rupture, peaking around day 7 and resolving after 2 weeks. The cerebral infarction associated with vasospasm contributes to poor outcomes, and therefore, a detailed understanding of the clinical presentation and management is essential. Initial recognition and management of SAH is found in Chapter 7, but because management of cerebral vasospasm is sufficiently specific in its approach, it warrants a separate simulation scenario.

THE PROBLEM BEFORE US

A common clinical presentation of DCI is a decline in the level or content of consciousness, although focal changes may come later. Patients may become restless, confused, drowsy, or withdrawn. The variety of clinical presentations and the frequent presence of other consciousness-altering physiologic derangements (e.g., fever, hyponatremia, and delirium) are obstacles to making a certain diagnosis of DCI. Key to its recognition are the following: (1) anticipation in high-risk patients, (2) considering the timing with onset day 3–10 following aneurysm rupture, and most importantly (3) assuming DCI until proven otherwise. High-risk patients include young people, active smokers, drug users, patients with poor clinical grade at presentation,[4] and patients with thick cisternal or ventricular clots on admission CT scan.[5] Many institutions use the modified Fisher scale to grade the amount of blood on CT scan,[6] which includes—next to scrutinizing cisternal blood—grading of intraventricular blood because it is considered an additional risk factor for cerebral vasospasm.[5,7]

Transcranial Doppler (TCD) ultrasonography is an accepted, widely used method to screen for or confirm vasospasm.[8] Cerebral vasospasm is suspected when the mean blood-flow velocity in the proximal segment of the middle cerebral artery (MCA) exceeds 120 cm/s. Cerebral vasospasm is considered severe when the velocity surpasses 200 cm/s. This velocity must be considered in the context of the extracranial internal carotid artery velocity (MCA/ICA ratio or Lindegaard ratio) to exclude hyperemia related to hypertension as the mechanism of the elevated intracranial velocity. Basilar artery vasospasm is suspected when the velocity in the artery exceeds 85 cm/s.[8,9]

CT angiogram can also demonstrate cerebral vasospasm, and CT perfusion may add diagnostic value, but may be more useful in the presence of focal deficits, where it may more directly influence treatment decisions. When DCI is diffuse, involving the bilateral cerebral hemispheres, cerebral blood flow is globally reduced and thus the cerebral perfusion study loses value as it relies on side-to-side comparison.

DCI should prompt rapid hemodynamic augmentation therapy, not to be confused with the so-called "triple H" (hypertension, hypervolemia, hemodilution) therapy. Both the hypervolemia and hemodilution components of "triple H" have limited efficacy and significant risks of fluid overload and myocardial demand resulting in myocardial ischemia. Thus, the medical management of DCI focuses on avoidance of hypovolemia and blood pressure augmentation using any vasopressor and subsequent assessment of neurologic function at each mean arterial blood pressure (MAP) level to determine the blood pressure value at which the patient's symptoms resolve.[2,10]

When patients cannot tolerate such an increase in MAP due to coronary ischemia or severe pulmonary edema or when sequential increases in the blood pressure do not lead to resolution of symptoms, endovascular options are considered. These include the intraarterial administration of calcium-channel antagonists such as verapamil (preferred in more diffuse or distal cerebral vasospasm), or angioplasty (appropriate in severe symptomatic cerebral vasospasm of the proximal segments). In most DCI management protocols, to avoid losing time, cerebral angiography is arranged while pursuing medical management.

As with any acute neurologic emergency, avoidance of hypoxemia, hyperthermia, and hypoglycemia, as well as positioning the head of the bed at 30 degrees, minimize secondary brain injury. In addition, studies in SAH have consistently found that fever independently correlates with poor outcome and that cerebral infarcts may be more common in patients with untreated fever.[11-13]

THE PRESENTING CLINICAL PROBLEM

A 70-year-old man presented with aneurysmal SAH (Fig. 8.1). He underwent successful coiling of a posterior circulation aneurysm. On worsening of the headache without change in the level of consciousness or restriction of vertical gaze, acute hydrocephalus was treated with lumbar drain placement (scheduled drainage of 10 cc every 2 h) with relief of headache. Neurologic examination remained normal throughout the hospital course with the exception of impaired short-term memory.

Now, on postrupture day 6, the patient is more confused and alternates between drowsiness and restlessness. Over a 12-h period, his MAP has gradually increased from 80 to 100 mm Hg, and he has been polyuric and febrile for several hours with no response to acetaminophen.

The learner must accomplish the following key competencies: (1) diagnose DCI; (2) ensure optimal oxygen, temperature, positioning, and cerebrospinal fluid diversion; (3) administer a fluid bolus and maintain an even fluid balance; (4) augment blood pressure; (5) check serum sodium and glucose; (6) assess response to augmentation; (7) augment blood pressure even more; (8) reassess response to augmentation; (9) escalate to cerebral angiogram when symptoms do not rapidly resolve; and (10) consider intraarterial administration of vasodilators or angioplasty (Fig. 8.2). Learning objectives are summarized in Table 8.1.

Preparation

The actor is placed in a hospital bed in the ED with a peripheral intravenous catheter inserted and vital signs showing on the monitor. Urinary catheterization is simulated by taping the tube to the bed near the actor's thigh. In the simulation package, learners will have the "Guidelines for the Management of Aneurysmal Subarachnoid Hemorrhage" to review in advance of the scenario.[1] Setup and required equipment are detailed in Table 8.2.

Coaching Actors

The actor receives instructions to appear awake (with eyes open) but inattentive to his environment. Specifically, he should limit eye contact and not follow instructions from the learner unless prompted repeatedly with simple commands such as "close your eyes" and "stick out your tongue." Intermittently, the actor should appear restless; for example, fidgeting with the blanket, repeatedly arching his back and extending both arms. These repetitive movements should be slow, nonpurposeful, and stereotyped. The actor is nonverbal.

The role of the ICU nurse is to act as the confederate. The nurse executes the learner's orders and serves as the conduit from facilitator to learner via headsets.

THE IDEAL LEARNER

The learner is aware the patient had a SAH and is in the neurosciences intensive care unit. On entering P's room, CONF introduces himself as the ICU nurse and states "he is becoming increasingly confused and agitated." CONF leads the learner to the CT scan (Fig. 8.1) to show the SAH. L clarifies the number of days since aneurysm rupture and progression of symptoms and learns that it is post-bleed day 6 and the changes have been gradual although P was normal at his last neuro check 2 h before. L notes the temperature

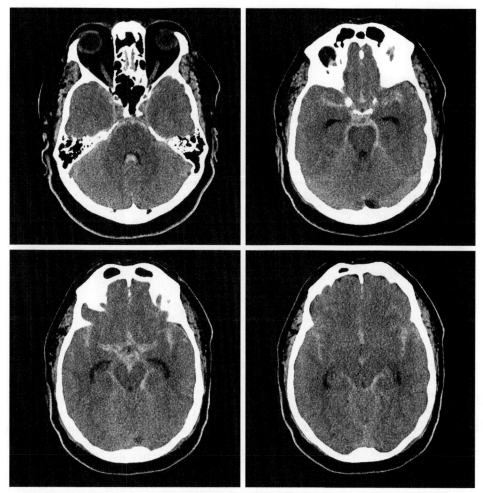

FIG. 8.1 CT scan of the brain showing diffuse subarachnoid blood within the bilateral cerebral convexities and extending into sylvian fissures and basal cisterns, along the tentorium. There is intraventricular hemorrhage within the fourth ventricle, and the temporal horns of the lateral ventricles are enlarged, consistent with acute hydrocephalus.

of 38.6°C, oxygen saturation of 91% on room air, MAP 99 mm Hg, and dilute urine in the catheter. On observation, he observes restlessness and repetitive stereotyped, purposeless movements. *P* is mute but follows some simple commands after repeated requests. *L* sees that *P*'s eyes move normally, face is symmetric, and all four limbs are moving against gravity with symmetry.

L asks *CONF* a series of questions—(1) "what is the fluid balance today?" (2) "how much urine has he been making per hour?" (3) "has the lumbar drain been functioning?"—and requests a chemistry panel, complete blood count, lactate, and cerebrospinal fluid analysis from the lumbar drain. *CONF* responds that

there has been a fluid deficit of 1.5 L since midnight, *P* has been making 200–300 cc urine/h, and that the drain is functioning well. *L* orders 1 L of normal saline, phenylephrine targeting a MAP of 110 mm Hg, oxygen by nasal cannula, and a cooling blanket to be placed underneath the patient. While *CONF* carries out these orders, *L* asks to review available TCD results and receives a printout of Table 8.3. *L* asks *CONF* whether the patient has received benzodiazepines or any other medications that could trigger delirium. *CONF* answers "no" and provides the laboratory results previously requested by *L*.

L reviews all results, paying particular attention to the glucose (normal), sodium, and cerebrospinal fluid

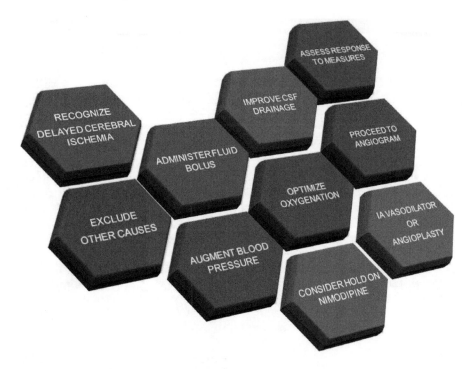

FIG. 8.2 Deconstructing key competencies in delayed cerebral ischemia.

TABLE 8.1
Objectives

- Develop a focused differential diagnosis for delayed deterioration after aneurysmal subarachnoid hemorrhage
- Diagnose delayed cerebral ischemia
- Provide adequate supportive care
- Recognize limitations of blood pressure augmentation
- Progress rationally from medical to neuroradiological intervention

---

gram stain (normal). Noting a serum sodium level of 132 mmol/L, *L* orders 0.2 mg fludrocortisone to be given twice daily. *L* notes a MAP of 112 mm Hg and proceeds to reexamine *P*. Finding him unchanged, *L* requests augmentation of the MAP to 120 mm Hg and tells CONF that the patient needs emergent cerebral angiography. *L* notices that *P* is less restless and that the unusual stereotyped movements have stopped. With a MAP of 130 mm Hg, *L* repeats the examination and finds *P* to be more attentive and verbal, although he remains visibly confused.

L is shown the angiography images on the monitor (Fig. 8.3). CONF asks "what do you think?" *L* describes diffuse vasospasm, worse in the left internal carotid, and basilar arteries. The facilitator calls the room and CONF answers. "It's the interventionalist—she wants to know what you want her to do." *L* proposes injection of intraarterial verapamil to both internal carotid arteries and the right vertebral artery and recommends avoidance of angioplasty with the rationale that (1) the patient is demonstrating clinical evidence of diffuse and distal DCI and (2) given the patient's signs of improvement, the higher risk of angioplasty should be avoided. Scenario ends.

THE NOT-SO-IDEAL LEARNER

We have identified the following common missteps. If any of these possible variations occur, the trainers can decide to end the simulation scenario.

1. *Learner does not recognize delayed cerebral ischemia.* Considering delirium, nonconvulsive seizures, hydrocephalus, or possibly feeling totally clueless, the learner becomes flustered. When this occurs, learners tend to go through a broad differential diagnosis, forgetting to consider the clinical context. This

TABLE 8.2
Scenario Setup for Delayed Cerebral Ischemia

People needed	• Simulation technician to control the monitor • Actor to play the intensive care unit nurse • Actor to play the patient • Attending physician or neurocritical care fellow to facilitate
Equipment needed	• Syringes • BP cuff and arterial line • IV line and saline bag • Oxygen by nasal cannula • Phenylephrine, norepinephrine, lorazepam, normal saline • Foley catheter with CritiCore • Lumbar drain kit • Laboratory results • Transcranial Doppler study results (Table 8.3)
Setup needed	• Monitor showing sinus rhythm, hypertension, mild hyperthermia, normal respiratory rate, and mild hypoxemia on room air • CT and cerebral angiography images on monitor (monitor turned off until learner requests imaging) (Figs. 8.1 and 8.3) • Foley catheter taped to bed with bladder temperature probe set to 38.6 C • Lumbar drain set up and taped to bed with xanthochromic colored fluid in bag

IV, intravenous catheter; *BP*, blood pressure.

postpones management of DCI and risks possible consequences of infarction.

2. *Learner diagnoses status epilepticus.* The presence of inattention and stereotyped movements without other focal deficits in the setting of mild hyponatremia leads some to conclude prematurely that nonconvulsive status epilepticus is responsible for the relatively acute deterioration. If they proceed to follow the SE treatment algorithm, their treatment choices may precipitate relative hypotension to the detriment of the patient.

3. *Learner considers rebleeding or hydrocephalus.* These options are not completely unreasonable. The learner may rush the patient to the CT scanner and call neurosurgery or attempt to drain extra cerebrospinal fluid as a therapeutic trial. These measures are unlikely to be harmful apart from delaying treatment of cerebral ischemia.

4. *Learner diagnoses delirium.* The learner attributes the changes to delirium given the patient's inattention and multiple risk factors including prolonged ICU stay, acute brain injury, mild hyponatremia, fever, and age. The learner focuses on treatment of fever, hyponatremia, evaluation for hospital-acquired infections, and may prescribe an antipsychotic drug.

5. *The learner does not consider endovascular options.* The learner continues to give fluid and augment blood pressure despite persistent neurologic deficits without first requesting catheter cerebral angiography, a failure that could lead to both cerebral infarction and myocardial ischemia.

ADAPTING THE SCENARIO

This case is written for senior neurology and neurosurgery residents. For neurocritical care fellows, easily able to navigate the case as written, medical complexity

TABLE 8.3
Transcranial Doppler Ultrasound

Date	Reading Type	ACA A1		ICA		MCA M1		PCA P1		BA	Units
		Right	Left	Right	Left	Right	Left	Right	Left		
PSAHD #2	Mean velocity	96	103	98	91	101	92	66	49	37	cm/s
PSAHD #4	Mean velocity	125	125	138	104	143	108	79	58		cm/s
PSAHD #6	Mean velocity	141	163	171	184	167	217		63	150	cm/s

ACA, anterior cerebral artery; *CA*, internal carotid artery; *cm/s*, centimeters/second; *PSAHD*, post-subarachnoid hemorrhage day; *MCA*, middle cerebral artery; *PCA*, posterior cerebral artery.

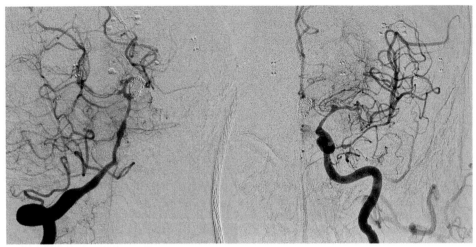

FIG. 8.3 Catheter cerebral angiography showing a coiled left superior cerebellar artery aneurysm and cerebral vasospasm in the vertebral (left) and left carotid (right) injections.

TABLE 8.4
Evidence for Treatment of Delayed Cerebral Ischemia[1]
• Transcranial Doppler monitoring is reasonable (class 2a, level of evidence B). Perfusion CT or MRI can be used to identify cerebral ischemia (class 2a, level of evidence B)
• Prophylactic cerebral angioplasty should not be used (high-quality evidence, strong recommendation).
• Induce hypertension in a stepwise fashion (moderate-quality evidence, strong recommendation)
• No specific inotropes/vasopressors recommended (moderate-quality evidence, strong recommendation)
• Intraarterial vasodilators and/or angioplasty may be considered, for ischemic symptoms refractory to medical management (moderate-quality evidence, strong recommendation)
• Balloon or pharmacologic angioplasty is reasonable for DCI without response to induced hypertension (class 2a, level of evidence B)

can be increased with the addition of coronary artery disease and ST elevation on the monitor during hemodynamic augmentation or inducing arrhythmias with vasopressors. Providing CT perfusion studies showing diffuse hypoperfusion and a normal angiogram suggesting diffuse distal vasospasm adds diagnostic complexity.

DEBRIEFING

Here we review the time course of complications following aneurysmal subarachnoid hemorrhage, clinical presentation of DCI, and its diagnosis.[14] A stepwise approach to treatment of DCI, which begins with blood pressure augmentation followed by endovascular therapy in those refractory to medical management, is reviewed and correction of hypovolemia emphasized. Debriefing can focus on three main discussion points. First, the variety of clinical presentations, including frequent odd stereotyped movements and restlessness, is described. Second, the guideline recommendations and level of evidence (not strong) can be reviewed. (Table 8.4). Third, the instructor should use this opportunity to discuss the dose and side effects of blood pressure—augmenting or vasodilating drugs (Table 8.5). The differential diagnosis can be reviewed and learners coached to prioritize possible DCI over other possibilities including delirium and nonconvulsive seizures.

TABLE 8.5
Blood Pressure Augmentation and Vasodilation

Norepinephrine	• Potent B-1 Agonist • Tachycardia • Hypoperfusion • Maximum infusion 3 mcg/kg/min
Vasopressin	• V_1 receptors for vasoconstriction • Reduced tachycardia • Maximum infusion 0.07 units/min
Dopamine	• Inotrope • More cardiac arrhythmias than norepinephrine • Maximum infusion 50 mcg/kg/min
Milrinone	• Phosphodiesterase inhibitor • Maximum infusion 1.25 mcg/kg/min

CONCLUSIONS

Simulating SAH should include its most important cause of secondary deterioration—cerebral vasospasm causing cerebral ischemia or infarctions. Simulating delayed cerebral ischemia offers learners the opportunity to diagnose and manage this challenging neurologic emergency firsthand with directed feedback. Actors can easily simulate the restlessness and inattention that is characteristic of delayed cerebral ischemia, and the scenario is easily adaptable for different learners.

REFERENCES

1. Connolly Jr ES, Rabinstein AA, Carhuapoma JR, et al. Guidelines for the management of aneurysmal subarachnoid hemorrhage: a guideline for healthcare professionals from the American Heart Association/American Stroke Association. *Stroke*. 2012;43:1711–1737.
2. Diringer MN, Bleck TP, Claude Hemphill 3rd J, et al. Critical care management of patients following aneurysmal subarachnoid hemorrhage: recommendations from the Neurocritical Care Society's Multidisciplinary Consensus Conference. *Neurocrit Care*. 2011;15:211–240.
3. Vergouwen MD, Vermeulen M, van Gijn J, et al. Definition of delayed cerebral ischemia after aneurysmal subarachnoid hemorrhage as an outcome event in clinical trials and observational studies: proposal of a multidisciplinary research group. *Stroke*. 2010;41:2391–2395.
4. Geraghty JR, Testai FD. Delayed cerebral ischemia after subarachnoid Hemorrhage: beyond vasospasm and towards a multifactorial pathophysiology. *Curr Atheroscler Rep*. 2017;19:50.
5. Claassen J, Bernardini GL, Kreiter K, et al. Effect of cisternal and ventricular blood on risk of delayed cerebral ischemia after subarachnoid hemorrhage: the Fisher scale revisited. *Stroke*. 2001;32:2012–2020.
6. Fisher CM, Kistler JP, Davis JM. Relation of cerebral vasospasm to subarachnoid hemorrhage visualized by computerized tomographic scanning. *Neurosurgery*. 1980;6:1–9.
7. Kramer AH, Hehir M, Nathan B, et al. A comparison of 3 radiographic scales for the prediction of delayed ischemia and prognosis following subarachnoid hemorrhage. *J Neurosurg*. 2008;109:199–207.
8. Sloan MA, Alexandrov AV, Tegeler CH, et al. Assessment: transcranial Doppler ultrasonography: report of the Therapeutics and Technology Assessment Subcommittee of the American Academy of Neurology. *Neurology*. 2004;62:1468–1481.
9. Sloan MA, Burch CM, Wozniak MA, et al. Transcranial Doppler detection of vertebrobasilar vasospasm following subarachnoid hemorrhage. *Stroke*. 1994;25:2187–2197.
10. Rabinstein AA, Lanzino G, Wijdicks EF. Multidisciplinary management and emerging therapeutic strategies in aneurysmal subarachnoid haemorrhage. *Lancet Neurol*. 2010;9:504–519.
11. Fernandez A, Schmidt JM, Claassen J, et al. Fever after subarachnoid hemorrhage: risk factors and impact on outcome. *Neurology*. 2007;68:1013–1019.
12. Naidech AM, Bendok BR, Bernstein RA, et al. Fever burden and functional recovery after subarachnoid hemorrhage. *Neurosurgery*. 2008;63:212–217.
13. Oliveira-Filho J, Ezzeddine MA, Segal AZ, et al. Fever in subarachnoid hemorrhage: relationship to vasospasm and outcome. *Neurology*. 2001;56:1299–1304.
14. Al-Mufti F, Amuluru K, Damodara N, El-Ghanem M, Nuoman R, Kamal N, Al-Marsoummi S, Morris NA, Dangayach NS, Mayer SA. Novel management strategies for medically-refractory vasospasm following aneurysmal subarachnoid hemorrhage. *J Neurol Sci*. 2018;15:44–51.

CHAPTER 9

Simulating Cerebral Venous Thrombosis

Few physicians consider a venous origin of an intracranial hemorrhage. Lobar-type hematomas usually are attributed to an underlying vascular malformation, amyloid angiopathy, or hypertension, but in younger individuals, particularly in females, thrombosis of the cerebral venous system should be considered. Cerebral venous thrombosis often has a multiday history of headaches followed later by focal neurologic signs or symptoms—a progression unlike arterial cerebral hemorrhage. Some of these symptoms are fleeting (e.g., paresthesias) or objectively hard to pinpoint (e.g., visual blurring), but the combination of a focused neurologic examination and appropriate neuroimaging will lead to the—nearly always somewhat surprising—discovery. The diagnosis can only be clearly established by CT venogram or MR venogram—and can be easily overlooked if no specific studies are ordered.

Moreover, there is a treatment paradox—anticoagulation in a patient with intracranial hemorrhage benefits the patient. This is because ongoing venous congestion leads to insufficient recruitment of collaterals and, eventually, a decrease in cerebral perfusion pressure, which leads to ischemia and intracranial hemorrhage. Any cerebral venous sinus occlusion can result in intracranial hemorrhages, which are basically hemorrhagic venous infarcts. Dural sinuses become involved and cause abnormalities of cerebrospinal circulation from decreased cerebrospinal fluid absorption. Eventually, venous congestion leads to increased intracranial pressure. This ongoing process, in which a developing venous clot propagates into the cortical branches or the larger superior sagittal sinus and leads to further venous infarction and hemorrhage, is the main rationale for treatment with anticoagulation. Mitigating propagation with anticoagulation will therefore also reduce development of infarction and hemorrhagic conversion.

Cerebral venous thrombosis—with a hemorrhagic infarct or expanding hematoma—may present with a variety of clinical features which include intractable headache as a result of increased intracranial pressure, focal clinical signs, or ophthalmoplegia with proptosis if the thrombosis is in the cavernous sinus. The recognition of this disorder remains difficult, and therefore, simulation of such a case benefits the learner by providing an opportunity to consider management options when suddenly confronted with this condition. For that reason, it is included in this book.

THE PROBLEM BEFORE US

Cerebral venous thrombosis is commonly associated with an underlying coagulopathy, although coagulation abnormalities might be difficult to find. Hereditary thrombophilia—and, particularly, Factor V Leiden thrombophilia or prothrombin GLY20210-ALA mutation—is the most commonly detected abnormality. In many patients, however, extensive evaluation does not yield a tangible result even after repeated testing.

Cerebral venous thrombosis is classically associated with pregnancy and the postpartum period in young females and is highly correlated with oral contraceptive use. Cancer is an unusual explanation in younger individuals but should be considered, particularly if there is prior evidence of other recent venous thromboembolic disease such as a deep venous thrombosis. Cerebral venous thrombosis is also a very unusual first presentation of cancer and occurs far more often in advanced terminal stages. A number of systemic or inflammatory diseases can be associated with cerebral venous thrombosis including systemic lupus erythematosus, antiphospholipid antibody syndrome, nephrotic syndrome, sarcoidosis, and myeloproliferative cancers. A seldom-considered cause of cerebral venous thrombosis is CSF hypotension, which causes traction in the venous system, sludging, and thrombosis (sometimes after a lumbar puncture). Cerebral venous thrombosis has been associated with high-altitude dehydration. However, these patients typically also have underlying thrombophilia, which is exacerbated by visiting high-altitude regions.[1-8] Head and neck infections and head trauma represent additional provoking factors, particularly in children.

Headache is the most common symptom of cerebral venous thrombosis, present in 89% of patients.[9] The onset of headache is usually gradual and progressive over several days, although some may present with a thunderclap headache or no headache at all.[10,11] Others have a more protracted course, which can result in long-standing headache, development of papilledema, decreased vision, and other nonspecific symptoms such as paresthesias or even brief episodes of weakness. Focal or more generalized seizures occur in approximately 20% of patients.[5] Seizures are seen far more often in patients with intracranial hemorrhage and usually occur before the diagnosis is made.

The diagnosis may not be apparent on a regular CT scan, which is normal in up to 30% of cases, and the findings that are present are frequently nonspecific.[1,7] A transverse sinus clot may appear as a string sign and less often in the falx, where recognition may be hampered by the common appearance of calcifications. Many patients present with what appears to be a small lobar hematoma. The radiologic characteristics often differ from a hypertensive lobar hemorrhage or from an arteriovenous malformation related hemorrhage in which the lesion contains a mixture of densities. No clear demarcation is seen with the hematoma as is usually apparent in arterial lobar hematomas. When the sagittal sinus is involved, bilateral or multifocal lesions can be seen due to involvement of multiple cortical branches. A CTV or MRV will establish the diagnosis and, in most patients, will initially show a clot in the transverse sinus. This may extend to the sagittal sinus, which immediately changes the urgency of the clinical picture.

Laboratory abnormalities are rarely present, although some patients may have evidence of dehydration with mild hypernatremia and increased hematocrit. Cerebral venous thrombosis can also be seen in the setting of bacterial meningitis, but then it is more focal and typically associated with mastoiditis (Chapter 15).

Cerebral venous thrombosis leads to dilatation of the venous and capillary bed followed by interstitial edema, disruption of veins, and formation of hematomas.

The venous system is most commonly obstructed at the transverse sinus extending to the superior sagittal sinus and eventually involving cortical veins. Internal cerebral vein or straight sinus occlusion may result in hemorrhagic infarction of the thalami or caudate nuclei. The treatment of cerebral venous thrombosis, as previously indicated, is, therefore, immediate initiation of anticoagulation with either low molecular-weight heparin (LMWH), or unfractionated heparin using a bolus and high intensity nomogram. LMWH and unfractionated heparin have been compared, and studies suggest that LMWH leads to better outcomes.[12,13] Anticoagulation in patients with an established intracranial hemorrhage will most likely cause some expansion of the hematoma. In some patients, anticoagulation may significantly enlarge the intracranial hematoma, causing mass effect. However, withholding heparin can result in new venous infarcts and hemorrhages and rapid worsening of the patient. Because some hemorrhages in the temporal lobe—occlusion of the vein of Labbé disrupts drainage of the temporal lobe and surrounding parenchyma of the sylvian fissure—can enlarge and become rapidly symptomatic, neurosurgeons should be involved; in some instances, they may have to proceed with urgent clot removal and decompressive craniectomy.[14,15] The likelihood of hemorrhage enlargement in patients who present with cerebral venous thrombosis and an associated hemorrhage, justifies initial management with unfractionated heparin, which allows more control as it can be easily reversed with protamine if surgery is required. Once the patient is adequately anticoagulated (usually within 24 h), and has not deteriorated clinically, heparin can be substituted for LMWH (LMWH does not have an effective antidote).

The general approach to more severe cases is to consider endovascular treatment, which would include catheterization of the jugular vein extending into the sagittal sinus, but only if the patient "fails" anticoagulation. However, in practice, many patients are insufficiently anticoagulated. Whether endovascular treatment is indicated as a first step is unresolved and, in general, discouraged. Endovascular lysis of the clot has been successful including in comatose patients with multiple hemorrhagic infarcts. A catheter is inserted via puncture of the jugular vein or through the transfemoral route, advanced to the transverse sinus, and, if possible, advanced to the superior sagittal sinus. Tissue-plasminogen activator is usually infused at 1 mg/h and may continue for up to 12 h or more depending on efficacy of clot lysis as determined by repeat angiography. The timing of endovascular thrombolysis is unresolved. We can expect increase in early endovascular intervention now that this option is readily available in many centers.

Long-term anticoagulation with warfarin is necessary if no cause is found; however, shorter periods can be considered if a precipitating etiology or risk factor has been identified and treated. Recanalization is very common in the first 6 months (up to 80% of documented cases).[16] A comparative clinical trial of dabigatran versus warfarin is underway, but practice may already have moved in that direction given the evidence that idarucizumab quickly reverses the anticoagulant effect of dabigatran and has been FDA approved.

THE PRESENTING CLINICAL PROBLEM

The patient is a 25-year-old woman who presented in the emergency department with intractable headaches, which she describes as thunderclap in onset 2 days ago, after her return from a trip to Machu Picchu. She describes feeling sick over the last couple of days with fatigue and frequent vomiting. The headache never fully subsided, although there has been some fluctuation in severity. She also describes blurred vision with some photophobia and sonophobia as well as a general feeling of lightheadedness. Her hearing is not affected. She has not had fevers or any other infectious symptoms. She uses oral contraceptives.

The learner should recognize the unusual presentation of the headache, elicit a history of a recent trip to a high-altitude region, obtain initial laboratory results with a finding of mild dehydration as a result of vomiting, identify oral contraceptives as a risk factor, and accurately interpret the CT scan. The main objectives of this scenario are (1) recognize headache characteristics of and risk factors for cerebral venous thrombosis; (2) identify venous hemorrhage on CT scan and proceed quickly with a CTV to diagnose the extent of the thrombosis; (3) initiate acute anticoagulation with appropriate intensity; (4) consider or, at least, discuss the possibility of endovascular management; and (5) consider the risk of enlargement of the hemorrhage, which might necessitate neurosurgical intervention. The objectives are summarized in Table 9.1; the key competencies are summarized in Fig. 9.1.

Preparation

An actor is placed in a hospital bed in the ED with a peripheral IV but normal vital signs including normal temperature, blood pressure, and heart rate. Before the simulation, learners receive the AHA/ASA Scientific Statement on the diagnosis and management of cerebral venous sinus thrombosis[7] to review in advance. The scenario setup is shown in Table 9.2.

Coaching Actors

Instructions for the actors are shown in Table 9.3. The actor is restless from the headache, complains of visual defect, and imitates an upper-quadrant visual field cut

TABLE 9.1 Objectives
• Recognize headache pattern and risk factors of cerebral venous thrombosis
• Identify venous hemorrhage on CT and produce a differential diagnosis
• Order appropriate neuroimaging to detect transverse sinus thrombosis
• Treat appropriately with high-intensity IV heparin
• Understand indications for endovascular thrombectomy

("pie in the sky" phenomenon). The actor will also report a tongue bite, suggesting a recent seizure.

THE IDEAL LEARNER

L enters and introduces herself to P and CONF after reading the ED Face Sheet. P will state that she has had significant intractable headaches since she returned from a trip and has been vomiting for the last couple of days. L elicits a history of thunderclap headache followed by persistent, milder headache with nausea and, more recently, blurred vision. She further identifies the tongue bite and the history of oral contraceptive use. L then performs a neurologic examination and finds a quadrantanopia. L orders laboratory studies including a chemistry panel, complete blood count, coagulation panel, and type and screen, as well as a CT scan, which shows the intracranial hemorrhage (Fig. 9.2A). CONF asks what caused the hemorrhage, and L provides a differential diagnosis of intracranial hemorrhage. L suggests that the patient may have a venous hemorrhage associated with cerebral venous thrombosis, given the headache characteristics hemorrhage location, and risk factor of oral contraceptive use. L orders a CTV or MRV to confirm the suspected diagnosis of cerebral venous thrombosis (Fig. 9.2B). L then reviews the laboratory studies and, concluding that they show evidence of dehydration, orders additional IV fluids. L decides to proceed with immediate anticoagulation with high-intensity heparin to prevent further worsening. L also orders 2 g of levetiracetam to prevent further seizures. L carefully considers the type of anticoagulation (heparin vs. LMWH) and explains to P the risk of further enlargement of the hematoma as well as the risk of not starting anticoagulation. L also considers the possibility of endovascular treatment if the patient does not improve and asks neurosurgery to weigh in and consider surgery if further enlargement or further swelling of the infarct is seen.

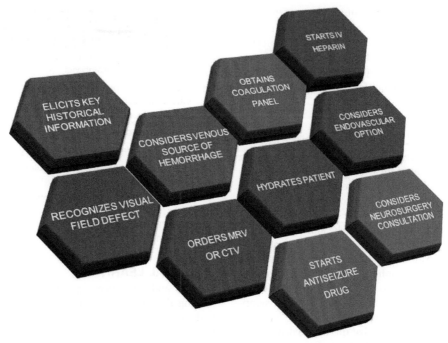

FIG. 9.1 Deconstructing key competencies in cerebral venous thrombosis.

TABLE 9.2 Scenario Setup for Cerebral Venous Thrombosis	
People needed	• Actor to play ED nurse • Actor to play patient • Attending physician or neurocritical care fellow to facilitate
Equipment needed	• ED Face Sheet with summary of the history • Laboratory results • Blood pressure cuff • IV line (18G IV in the antecubital fossa to facilitate CT venogram)
Setup needed	• Normal vital signs • Monitor showing BP 140/95 mmHg • Patient lying in bed (head of bed at 30°) • CT scan • CT venogram

TABLE 9.3 Actor Instructions Before Simulation
• Provide history of thunderclap headache
• Report that headache is still present; asks for emesis basin
• Show discomfort with headache: grab head frequently, appear restless
• Display a left quadrantanopia ("pie in the sky" type)
• If asked about bowel or bladder incontinence, muscle or mouth soreness, report waking up with mouth soreness this morning and finding you had bitten your tongue on the side
• Provide previous history of travel to high-altitude location

THE NOT-SO-IDEAL LEARNER

Cerebral venous sinus thrombosis remains a difficult-to-recognize diagnosis, and we can expect the following errors in judgment.

1. *The learner does not recognize that the hemorrhage might be of venous origin.* This is a common error and can lead to insufficient evaluation of the patient, withholding of anticoagulation, and propagation of the clot.
2. *The learner is unable to identify the cause of cerebral venous thrombosis.* In this case, the patient was dehydrated after a trip to a high-altitude region and

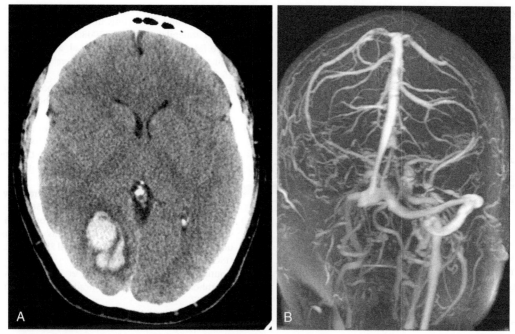

FIG. 9.2 **(A)** CT scan of the brain showing lobar hematoma in the right occipital lobe, **(B)** CT venogram showing occlusion of the right transverse sinus and internal jugular vein.

was predisposed by the use of oral contraceptive pills. The learner does not note that the patient is mildly dehydrated due to vomiting and fails to rehydrate the patient.

3. *The learner does not identify the tongue bite, a common finding in neurologic patients.* This is important because the lobar hematoma predisposes the patient to further seizures. Therefore, antiseizure drugs should be administered. This is particularly important because the patient will be fully anticoagulated, and uncontrolled seizures may potentially harm the patient.

4. *The learner does not consider IV heparin.* This is the main issue, and high-intensity IV heparin is needed to avoid propagation of the clot despite it being a hemorrhage.

5. *The learner does not consider endovascular options.* Endovascular options are often considered but not pursued. Worsening despite adequate anticoagulation is an indication for endovascular intervention.

ADAPTING THE SCENARIO

The scenario can be made more challenging by removing the focal deficits and providing a normal head CT scan. This is not an uncommon presentation, and the combination of progressive headache and a risk factor for venous sinus thrombosis should prompt the learner to perform a lumbar puncture, which will reveal a high opening pressure (sometimes the only clue). Further complications might include the addition of clinical worsening due to progressive cerebral edema, which would require hypertonic saline (as mannitol could be dehydrating) and consideration of escalation to hemicraniectomy.

DEBRIEFING

Debriefing of this clinical diagnosis is important because it allows the possibility to discuss several key issues in acute neurology. First, it is important to discuss the differential diagnosis of intracranial hemorrhage, particularly when it pertains to a lobar hematoma. Emphasizing that a hemorrhage could be of venous origin is important. The discussion can also be extended toward the conditions associated with cerebral venous thrombosis and how best to evaluate and assess their severity (Table 9.4). Debriefing can also include the indications for endovascular management and the difficulties of deciding when to proceed. Finally, the debriefing can emphasize the need for a high index of

TABLE 9.4
Common Considerations With Cerebral Venous Thrombosis

- Congenital hematologic conditions
- Pregnancy and puerperium
- Dehydration
- Traumatic brain injury
- Cerebral hypotension syndrome
- Oral contraceptives
- Estrogens
- Glucocorticoids
- Connective tissue and inflammatory diseases
- Head and neck infections
- Malignancy

suspicion given frequently normal neuroimaging and the absolute necessity of high-intensity anticoagulation, even in the presence of intracerebral hemorrhage, to prevent further propagation of the clot.

CONCLUSIONS

Cerebral venous thrombosis and intracranial hemorrhage are well suited to simulation. The intractable headache, evidence of undetected seizures, as well as clear additional neuroimaging showing a clot in the cerebral venous system, can all be easily incorporated into a simple scenario. This condition is rarely seen, but the urgency is evident, particularly if anticoagulation is delayed.

REFERENCES

1. Bousser MG, Chiras J, Bories J, et al. Cerebral venous thrombosis—a review of 38 cases. *Stroke.* 1985;16: 199–213.
2. Cantu C, Barinagarrementeria F. Cerebral venous thrombosis associated with pregnancy and puerperium. Review of 67 cases. *Stroke.* 1993;24:1880–1884.
3. Dentali F, Poli D, Scoditti U, et al. Long-term outcomes of patients with cerebral vein thrombosis: a multicenter study. *J Thromb Haemost.* 2012;10:1297–1302.
4. Ferro JM, Canhao P, Bousser MG, et al. Early seizures in cerebral vein and dural sinus thrombosis: risk factors and role of antiepileptics. *Stroke.* 2008;39:1152–1158.
5. Ferro JM, Correia M, Rosas MJ, et al. Seizures in cerebral vein and dural sinus thrombosis. *Cerebrovasc Dis.* 2003; 15:78–83.
6. Riva N, Ageno W. Approach to thrombosis at unusual sites: splanchnic and cerebral vein thrombosis. *Vasc Med.* 2017;22:529–540.
7. Saposnik G, Barinagarrementeria F, Brown Jr RD, et al. Diagnosis and management of cerebral venous thrombosis: a statement for healthcare professionals from the American Heart Association/American Stroke Association. *Stroke.* 2011;42:1158–1192.
8. Silvis SM, de Sousa DA, Ferro JM, et al. Cerebral venous thrombosis. *Nat Rev Neurol.* 2017;13:555–565.
9. Ferro JM, Canhao P, Stam J, et al. Prognosis of cerebral vein and dural sinus thrombosis: results of the International Study on Cerebral Vein and Dural Sinus Thrombosis (ISCVT). *Stroke.* 2004;35:664–670.
10. Coutinho JM, Stam J, Canhao P, et al. Cerebral venous thrombosis in the absence of headache. *Stroke.* 2015;46: 245–247.
11. de Bruijn SF, Stam J, Kappelle LJ. Thunderclap headache as first symptom of cerebral venous sinus thrombosis. CVST Study Group. *Lancet.* 1996;348:1623–1625.
12. Coutinho J, de Bruijn SF, Deveber G, et al. Anticoagulation for cerebral venous sinus thrombosis. *Cochrane Database Syst Rev.* 2011:CD002005.
13. Misra UK, Kalita J, Chandra S, et al. Low molecular weight heparin versus unfractionated heparin in cerebral venous sinus thrombosis: a randomized controlled trial. *Eur J Neurol.* 2012;19:1030–1036.
14. Aaron S, Alexander M, Moorthy RK, et al. Decompressive craniectomy in cerebral venous thrombosis: a single centre experience. *J Neurol Neurosurg Psychiatry.* 2013;84: 995–1000.
15. Zuurbier SM, Coutinho JM, Majoie CB, et al. Decompressive hemicraniectomy in severe cerebral venous thrombosis: a prospective case series. *J Neurol.* 2012;259: 1099–1105.
16. Ferro JM, Dentali F, Coutinho JM, et al. Rationale, design, and protocol of a randomized controlled trial of the safety and efficacy of dabigatran etexilate versus dose-adjusted warfarin in patients with cerebral venous thrombosis. *Int J Stroke.* 2018;13:766–770.

CHAPTER 10

Simulating Coma of Unknown Cause

The cause of acute coma is usually obvious upon review of a head CT scan. Acute coma in a patient with a normal, noncontrast head CT scan is arguably the most disconcerting clinical situation encountered in neurology. It requires a methodical approach, an understanding of the conditions that may present in this manner, their respective probabilities, and possible consequences of delay in diagnosis. Emergency physicians may already have an inkling of a possible intoxication, and many patients found by emergency medical services may already have had a fingerstick glucose performed. The list of potential causes, however, is vast and includes several categories including seizures, infection, anoxic-ischemic brain injury, and acute metabolic diseases. Conditions such as fulminant bacterial meningitis may lead to irreversible neurologic disability or death if there is a delay in treatment (Chapter 15), while more common causes such as drug intoxication may recover spontaneously with time—although not always (e.g., heroin). A thorough understanding of the differential diagnosis can assist the physician in prioritizing diagnostic testing and initiating empiric therapies. Typically, physicians faced with a patient with coma of unknown cause will ensure airway patency, effective ventilation and hemodynamic stability, optimize physiology to prevent secondary brain injury, and promptly treat readily identifiable reversible causes (e.g., hypoglycemia). However, they also must empirically treat possible causes such as brain infection, or reverse opioid intoxication with naloxone.

Simulation provides novice physicians with an environment in which to experience the significant uncertainty that the provider feels when faced with a "CT-negative coma" and offers advanced learners an opportunity to hone their approach. We have found that most learners do appreciate the experience of going through a systematic thought process. Many learners will recognize a number of reversible causes of coma and develop a strategy for establishing an early diagnosis.

THE PROBLEM BEFORE US

Coma is defined by unresponsiveness to external stimuli. The patient's eyes may open to pain, or there may be no eye opening. There should be no fixation or tracking, and the best motor response is that of withdrawal to pain. Brainstem reflexes may be preserved, or they may be partially absent.[1] Knowing the structures that are responsible for an awake state (the ascending neuronal networks from the brainstem and thalamus that project to the cortex), coma localizes to one of three locations: the bilateral cerebral hemispheres (cortex or white matter), bilateral thalami, or brainstem.[2]

Traditionally, one expects the neurologic examination to provide sufficient clues to amalgamate into a probable diagnosis, but neurologic examination in a patient with a normal CT scan often yields few localizing findings. Small pupils could point to a pontine infarction (not yet seen on CT scan) or indicate an opioid overdose (currently, the most common culprits are fentanyl, carfentanyl, or heroin). Dilated pupils might signal drugs with a marked sympathetic drive such as cocaine or tricyclic antidepressants. Some patients will have a focality identifiable on examination, which we can expect to see in cerebrovascular causes of coma including basilar artery occlusion, acute thalamic and brainstem stroke, deep cerebral venous sinus thrombosis, or posterior reversible vasoconstriction syndrome.[3] Examples include anisocoria, skew deviation, and spontaneous nystagmus. A useful initial approach is redundant; "initially" conveys same meaning to assess whether the patient has brainstem signs (e.g., nystagmus, anisocoria, absent corneal reflexes, extensor posturing). Positive brainstem signs should immediately prompt a CT angiogram (CTA) to diagnose a basilar artery embolus, which then needs immediate endovascular retrieval (lack of a visible clot on CT does not rule out this diagnosis). Even with a normal CTA, an MRI might still reveal lesions in the thalami or brainstem responsible for coma.[3]

Patients with a central nervous system (CNS) infection or nonconvulsive status epilepticus do not typically present with focal deficits. Moreover, poisoning, drug toxicity, and acute metabolic derangements (except hypoglycemia, diabetic ketoacidosis, and nonketotic hyperglycemia), do not present with focal deficits but mostly a change in muscle tone—flaccidity or spasticity.

Additional help may come from abnormal laboratory findings, many of which are related to intoxication (e.g., hyperammonemia associated with acetaminophen overdose). Blood gas analysis may provide some clues when there is a metabolic acidosis (e.g., atypical alcohol ingestion, salicylate overdose), anion gap metabolic acidosis (e.g., cyanide), or increased osmolar gap (methanol and ethylene glycol). [1]

Other pertinent questions include the following. Is the patient intoxicated (self-inflicted or accidental)? Is there a CNS infection (Herpes simplex encephalitis or fulminant bacterial meningitis)? Is the patient actively seizing (nonconvulsive status epilepticus) or markedly postictal? Does the patient need hormone replacement (e.g., hypothyroidism, Addison's disease)?[4–6]

This scenario teaches the recognition of severe hypothyroidism. Myxedema coma is rare but should be considered in any comatose patient with hypothermia, respiratory acidosis, hyponatremia, or a combination of these.[7] Patients with poorly controlled hypothyroidism and a precipitating event (such as infection, cold exposure, myocardial infarction, or intake of sedatives or opioids) are at highest risk. Patients variably present with altered mental status, hypothermia, decompensated heart failure, kidney, or respiratory failure.[8] The clinical examination of myxedematous coma provides sufficient clues[8]—but only if all the dots are connected. There are many depressed ("hypo") features: bradycardia, hypoventilation,[9] hypothermia, and hypodynamic precordium. Laboratory findings may also show hypoxemia and hyponatremia. If an electroencephalogram (EEG) is obtained, brain waves are hypoactive (diffuse slowing). Periorbital edema can occur, but more commonly, the patient develops nonpitting edema in the extremities. Many patients have experienced substantial hair loss.[10] The diagnosis is based on low T_4 and elevated TSH levels. Decreased gluconeogenesis may lead to hypoglycemia.[7] Management consists of admission to an intensive care unit for ventilatory and hemodynamic support and thyroid hormone replacement.

THE PRESENTING CLINICAL PROBLEM

A 62-year-old woman presents after her husband found her unresponsive in bed in the morning and called 911. Paramedics found her in bed with bradycardia and hypoventilation; she was intubated with succinylcholine and no sedation.

The patient lives at home with her husband, who noticed that she was very tired and confused the evening before presentation. Specifically, she repeated questions and wandered aimlessly around the house. For the past week, she seemed to have slowed responses. Medical history includes hypertension, hyperlipidemia, hypothyroidism, and chronic back pain. She is a former smoker but does not drink alcohol or use illicit drugs. On review of systems, she has been generally fatigued for the past several weeks without fevers, chills, or weight loss, but she has had increased back pain, for which she was given oxycodone 2 weeks ago. Her routine medications were refilled 3 weeks ago; she is compliant with her medication regimen. On examination, her eyes are closed and do not open to voice or pain. Pupillary, corneal, oculocephalic, cough, and gag responses are present. There is no localization to pain, but there is a delayed, slow, symmetric withdrawal in all extremities. The head CT scan is normal.

The main objectives are to (1) obtain the critical components of the history and perform a coma examination; (2) direct the diagnostic evaluation, prioritizing treatable causes; (3) diagnose myxedema coma; (4) discount opioids as main cause for coma with naloxone; and (5) review CT scan and decide if it is normal (Table 10.1). The key competencies of the scenario are summarized in Fig. 10.1.

Preparation

The mannequin is placed in a hospital bed in the ED with a peripheral IV inserted and vital signs showing on the monitor. Two weeks before the simulation, learners receive a book chapter on the approach to the comatose patient to review in advance of the scenario. Additional setup and equipment required are detailed in Table 10.2.

TABLE 10.1
Objectives

- Complete a thorough and efficient history and coma examination.
- Direct the diagnostic evaluation of coma of unknown cause.
- Prioritize treatable causes in the diagnostic evaluation.
- Diagnose myxedema coma.
- Improve knowledge of the differential diagnosis of acute 'CT-negative coma.'
- Develop an algorithmic approach to the acutely comatose patient.

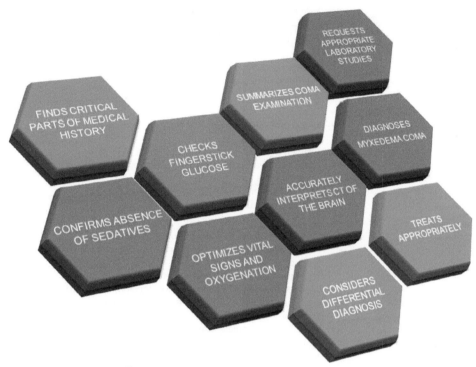

FIG. 10.1 Deconstructing key competencies in coma of unknown cause.

Coaching Actors

The actor portraying the spouse provides information requested by the learner. The actor's script lists all relevant history of present illness, past medical and social history, review of systems, and medications. The actor should answer "no" to any question for which the answer is not provided in the script. After the learner has taken a history and examined the patient, the actor asks, "What do you think is going on? Is my wife going to be okay?"

The ED nurse acts as the confederate in this scenario, answering questions about the prehospital and emergency department care before the learner's arrival, describing the examination in response to the learner's maneuvers, administering medications, ordering studies as requested, and providing results at the direction of the facilitator. Instructions to the actor and confederate are summarized in Table 10.3.

THE IDEAL LEARNER

L enters *P*'s room and introduces herself to *CONF* and *P*'s husband. *L* immediately sees the vital signs on the monitor, taking particular note of the hypothermia, and efficiently takes a focused, relevant medical history from the patient's spouse by quickly eliciting information about symptoms, evolution and timeline of events, recent exposures or illnesses, past medical history, and associated pertinent positive and negative symptoms on review of systems. She then reviews *P*'s medication list.

L inquiries about medications and fluids administered in the field and the emergency department and recommends head-of-the-bed elevation to 30 degrees, IV crystalloids, and pressors as needed to support a mean arterial pressure of ≥ 65 mmHg. She requests a STAT fingerstick glucose. When *CONF* reports that it is 65 mg/dL, she requests that 500 mg IV thiamine be given followed by 1 amp of D50. *L* performs a focused examination and, finding no changes in pupils and reactivity or eye movements, localizes coma to the bilateral cerebral hemispheres. She requests a large number of laboratory studies listed in Table 10.4, head CT scan, and empiric administration of dexamethasone, vancomycin, ceftriaxone, ampicillin, and acyclovir (after noting the hypothermia). *CONF* directs *L* to the monitor showing the CT scan (completed on arrival), which she correctly interprets as normal.

When asked by the spouse what is going on and whether his wife will get better, *L* answers the questions

TABLE 10.2
Scenario Setup for Coma of Unknown Cause

People needed	• Actor to play the emergency department nurse • Actor to play the patient's spouse • Attending or neurocritical care fellow to facilitate
Equipment needed	• 2 headsets (emergency physician, facilitator) • Syringes • Blood pressure cuff • Intravenous catheter • Oxygen by nasal cannula • Naloxone, lorazepam, ceftriaxone, vancomycin, acyclovir, ampicillin, D50, thiamine, normal saline • Mechanical ventilator • Laboratory results

Setup needed	• SimMan 3G on hospital bed
	  • Pupils reactive and blink shut off (eyes closed)
	  • BP cuff, ECG leads, pulse oximetry, peripheral IV ×2 attached
	  • Intubated
	  • Catheterized with Foley catheter
	• Monitor showing sinus rhythm, hypotension, bradycardia, hypothermia, low respiratory rate, and normal oxygenation on room air
	• Wrap legs to simulate edema
	• Normal head CT on monitor (monitor turned off until learner requests imaging)

IV, intravenous catheter; *BP*, blood pressure; *SpO2*, peripheral capillary oxygen saturation.

TABLE 10.3
Instructions to Actors Before Simulation

• Simulated patient is a mannequin, which allows portrayal of marked changes in vital signs.
• Spouse provides short history of malaise and fatigue but also hair loss (patient recently purchased a wig).
• Nurse is present to guide and obtain test results but may ask prodding questions about the diagnosis.
• Nurse will explain that extremities are swollen.

quickly and effectively, explaining that they need to work quickly to identify the cause in case it requires rapid treatment. At this stage, *l* is considering a differential diagnosis of (1) opiate overdose, (2) meningoencephalitis, (3) sepsis, (4) nonconvulsive status epilepticus, or, although rare, (5) myxedema coma (given her history of hypothyroidism and recent increase in opioid dose). *l* requests administration of IV naloxone, 0.4 mg, to be repeated every 2 min if no response. When 10 mg has been administered with no response, she concludes that the coma did not result from opioid toxicity. She orders an emergent EEG and inquires after the previously requested

laboratory results. *l* carefully reviews the laboratory results and notes significant elevation of the thyroid-stimulating hormone level. Free T3 and T4 values are pending.

Quickly synthesizing the information she has collected (i.e., female patient with hypothyroidism presenting with acute coma, hypotension, bradycardia, hypothermia, and a plausible precipitant [opioid increase]), *l* diagnoses myxedema coma, recommends passive rewarming, blood pressure support, frequent glucose monitoring, admission to the medical intensive care unit, and consultation with endocrinology for management. However, due to the urgency of the

TABLE 10.4 Key Laboratory Tests	
Complete blood Count	Normal
Chemistry panel	
• Sodium	131 (135–145 mmol/L)
• Potassium	4 (3.2–5 mmol/L)
• Chloride	102 (98–107 mmol/L)
• Glucose	71 (70–140 mg/dL)
• Bicarbonate	30 (22–29 mmol/L)
• Blood urea nitrogen	28 (8–24 (mg/dL)
• Creatinine	0.6 (0.8–1.3 mg/dL)
• Calcium	9.1 (8.9–10.1 mg/dL)
Arterial blood gas	Normal
Troponin	Normal
Liver function tests including ammonia	Normal
Thyroid-stimulating hormone	106 (0.3–4.2 mIU/L)
Troponin	Normal
Lactate	Normal
Creatine Kinase	300 (38–176 U/L)
Blood alcohol level	Negative
Urine drug screen	Positive for opiates
Urinalysis	Normal

TABLE 10.5 Classification of Coma

Structural brain injury
- Hemisphere with mass effect
- Bilateral hemispheres
- Cerebellum with mass effect
- Brainstem

Acute toxic-metabolic-endocrine derangement
- Sodium abnormalities
- Glucose abnormalities
- Liver failure
- Renal failure
- Hypercapnia
- Hyperammonemia
- Hypothyroidism

Diffuse physiologic brain dysfunction
- Seizures
- Poisoning
- Drug use
- Hypothermia

Psychogenic unresponsiveness
- Acute catatonia
- Malingering

situation, a loading dose of 200 mcg T_4 IV is warranted, typically followed by oral replacement later (1.6 mcg/kg). Scenario ends.

THE NOT-SO-IDEAL LEARNER

We have identified the following common missteps.

1. *The learner does not prioritize potentially fatal causes.* The learner considers a broad differential diagnosis and gets lost in her own maze. The learner directs a thorough investigation but does not consider the relative urgency of the possibilities leading to delays in excluding hypoglycemia, CNS infection, and nonconvulsive status epilepticus.

2. *The learner overinterprets CT scan.* Some learners attribute significance to artefactual or incidental findings. They may have difficulty changing focus when the provided—completely normal—CT scan does not indicate a clear-cut cause for coma. This scenario also teaches learners that some tests can be unexpectedly normal and they may have to change course.

3. *The learner does not consider drugs or paralytics.* Perhaps the most common etiologies of acute coma are toxic and metabolic in nature. Drugs must therefore be considered whenever a patient presents with acute coma, no localizing findings on examination, and normal head CT. Failure to consider drugs leads to unnecessary testing in patients with drug-induced coma.

4. *The learner ignores secondary brain insults.* Irrespective of the primary injury-inducing mechanism, the brain can sustain secondary injury through hypotension, hypoxemia, hyperthermia, or hypoglycemia. This patient was mechanically ventilated and hypothermic; however, head-of-the-bed elevation, early exclusion of hypoglycemia, and blood pressure support were indicated.

5. *The learner ignores significance of vital sign derangements.* Hypotension, bradycardia, and hypothermia are helpful clues to possible etiologies in the differential diagnosis. Given the elevated thyroid-stimulating hormone, these findings clinch the diagnosis.

ADAPTING THE SCENARIO

The purpose of this scenario is to afford learners the experience of navigating the evaluation of an acutely comatose patient with normal neuroimaging. However,

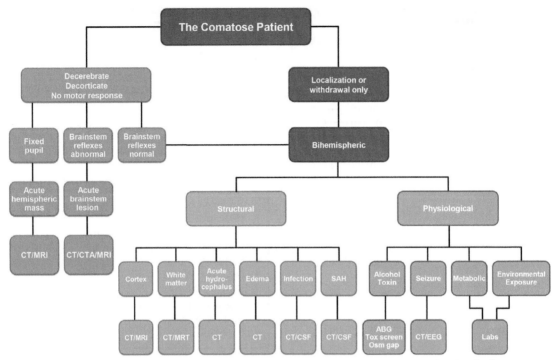

FIG. 10.2 The differential diagnosis of coma and approach using clinical and neuroimaging findings.

many other diagnoses achieve the same objectives (e.g., opioid overdose, carbon monoxide poisoning, or nonconvulsive status epilepticus). This scenario is designed for relatively novice learners and is applicable to all practitioners of hospital medicine. With only slight adaptation, different learners can still achieve the major objective of developing an approach to the patient with acute coma of unknown cause.

DEBRIEFING

The primary focus of the debrief is to guide the learner to develop a strategy for patients with coma of unknown cause and a normal brain CT scan. We review the importance of considering the history, localization, frequency of potential etiologies, and prioritization of treatable causes in the development of a diagnostic plan. Table 10.5 provides a useful template for discussion. Fig. 10.2 can be used to discuss systematically the step-by-step process of narrowing the causes to achieve a resolution and diagnosis. Learners often begin with a very wide differential diagnosis and have difficulty narrowing it. Myxedema coma is admittedly uncommon, and most reports are single case reports emphasizing the difficulty with its recognition.[11-13]

CONCLUSIONS

A comatose patient with a normal CT scan and no known trigger or other obvious circumstance can rattle even the most experienced physician. Preparation and practice in the development and execution of an algorithmic approach to the diagnostic evaluation of this condition facilitates rapid diagnosis and treatment of reversible causes. Our scenario of an endocrine emergency systematically merges clinical and laboratory findings in a patient with little or no neurologic findings other than deep unresponsive coma.

REFERENCES

1. Wijdicks EF. The bare essentials: coma. *Pract Neurol.* 2010; 10:51–60.
2. Merchut MP. Approach to the comatose patient. In: Biller J, ed. *Practical Neurology.* Philadelphia: Wolters Kluwer; 2017:52–58.
3. Edlow JA, Rabinstein A, Traub SJ, Wijdicks E. Diagnosis of reversible causes of coma. *Lancet.* 2014;384:2064–2076.
4. Akamizu T, Satoh T, Isozaki O, et al. Diagnostic criteria, clinical features, and incidence of thyroid storm based on nationwide surveys. *Thyroid.* 2012;22:661–679.
5. Dutta P, Bhansali A, Masoodi SR, et al. Predictors of outcome in myxedema coma: a study from a tertiary care center. *Crit Care.* 2008;12:R1.

6. Mathew V, Misgar RA, Ghosh S, et al. Myxedema coma: a new look into an old crisis. *J Thyroid Res*. 2011;2011:493462.

7. Kwaku MP, Burman KD. Myxedema coma. *J Intensive Care Med*. 2007;22:224–231.

8. Klubo-Gwiezdzinska J, Wartofsky L. Thyroid emergencies. *Med Clin North Am*. 2012;96:385–403.

9. Zwillich CW, Pierson DJ, Hofeldt FD, et al. Ventilatory control in myxedema and hypothyroidism. *N Engl J Med*. 1975;292:662–665.

10. Heymann WR. Cutaneous manifestations of thyroid disease. *J Am Acad Dermatol*. 1992;26:885–902.

11. Fjølner J, Søndergaard E, Kampmann U, Nielsen S. Complete recovery after severe myxoedema coma complicated by status epilepticus. *BMJ Case Rep*. March 25, 2015;83.

12. Gish DS, Loynd RT, Melnick S, Nazir S. Myxoedema coma: a forgotten presentation of extreme hypothyroidism. *BMJ Case Rep*. June 28, 2016. pii: bcr2016216225.

13. Garrahy A, Agha A. Dementia, cardiomyopathy and pseudo-obstruction in a 63-year-old female. *Eur J Intern Med*. 2018;55:e5–e6.

CHAPTER 11

Simulating Neuromuscular Respiratory Failure

Many patients enter emergency departments with shortness of breath. Very few of these patients will have a primary neurological cause for their respiratory failure, and if they do, its cause is known and part of anticipated disease progression. Typically, these emergency department admissions have already been diagnosed with amyotrophic lateral sclerosis or previously been treated for myasthenia gravis. These patients are weak or getting weaker and cannot breathe well, at which point they must visit the emergency department. The diagnostic challenges are to recognize that the respiratory failure is neuromuscular in origin and then to sort out whether the neuromuscular respiratory failure requires ventilator assistance. Weakness from neuromuscular disease has recognized clinical characteristics, and many manifest as mechanical failure.

We chose worsening myasthenia gravis as a representative example of neuromuscular respiratory failure and its immediate important consequences, designated with the predictive moniker *myasthenic crisis*.[1,2] This also allows us to prod the learner for basic knowledge of management with immunomodulation therapies, discuss the noninvasive mechanical ventilation options, and showcase the decision-making process regarding intubation in this condition, so different from others.[3] Every emergency room physician knows that lackadaisical admission of these patients with minimal findings to a regular hospital ward could lead to worsening—even when seemingly stable—and a call to the rapid-response team who might have to manage respiratory (and circulatory) arrest.

Teaching with videotapes of patients with neuromuscular respiratory failure is instructive, but in our experience, simulation of respiratory failure has also been quite feasible. This is because the manifestations of neuromuscular respiratory failure can be easily teased out and taught, and many of the clinical features can be effortlessly imitated by most actors. Simulation of acute neuromuscular failure in myasthenia gravis focuses on priorities in management rather than a close imitation of clinical symptoms.

THE PROBLEM BEFORE US

Knowledge of the basic facts about the major components of mechanical respiratory failure requires insight into the anatomy of the muscles of inspiration. The main muscle of inspiration is the diaphragm, and its recruitment creates a tremendous force and torque, necessary to lengthen the chest cavity and elevate the ribs. As a result, air moves in, but this also depends on the inspiratory pressure at peak expiration, the resistance of the chest wall, and health of lung and parenchyma—and each may act as a counter force preventing good air in-flow.[4-11] The diaphragm is innervated by the phrenic nerve, which originates in the mid- and high cervical regions from C3 to C5.

Expiration, on the other hand, is passive and a result of recoiling with typically inactive abdominal muscles, but contraction can increase intra-abdominal pressure and further elevate the diaphragm when expiration needs to be more forceful. Its function is also needed for coughing to clear the main airways, perhaps just as important as adequate inspiration. Adequate respiratory mechanics require flexibility of movement and an intact chest wall. Of course, inspiration as a result of diaphragmatic contraction is coordinated with upper-airway musculature, including an open pharynx and larynx, and is fully synchronous with diaphragmatic contraction.

Most diaphragm muscle failure stems from acute neuromuscular disorders, but given the full anatomic trajectory, weakness may also develop from a spinal cord lesion or from the brainstem. The nucleus ambiguus is responsible for dilating the muscles of the soft palate, pharynx, and larynx—this cluster of neurons provides an open, unobstructed airway. One can, therefore, imagine that acute brainstem lesions can result in both bulbar and diaphragmatic weakness if the lesion extends into the high cervical region.[12]

Neuromuscular respiratory failure can first present with subtle findings, such as when the patient has only shallow, rapid breathing, and halting speech, before appearing noticeably uncomfortable. Pulse oximetry may not show hypoxemia, and the arterial blood gas can be within normal limits until late in the course of respiratory failure. Nevertheless, the patient has shortness of breath and, often, a sensation of not being able to catch a full breath.[13] This eventually progresses to far more dramatic presentations in which the patient becomes tachypneic, tachycardic, and starts pooling secretions from inability to swallow them. At that time, patients are dysphonic and hoarse. Many of these patients also display restlessness, a reluctance to lie down, and feel most comfortable sitting upright. They may be anxious and, sometimes, obviously panicked. On examination, they have a mild sinus tachycardia with a heart rate of more than 100 beats/min, slight tachypnea with a rate of more than 20 breaths/min, and may be using accessory muscles such as the sternocleidomastoid or scalene muscles. Because the patient is unable to create large tidal volumes, speech is halting, creating a staccato-type delivery (this is a comparable sound to trying to speak after expiration). On further examination, the patient may have weakness of the oropharyngeal muscles and might actually be using the accessory muscles. Palpating these muscles, such as the sternocleidomastoid, might demonstrate contraction. Often unrecognized is a thoracoabdominal dyssynchrony, where there is a to-and-fro, rocking-horse movement with some breaths. It is more definitively apparent if the patient is placed in a supine position.

A few additional tests are available in the emergency department or intensive care unit. Pulmonary function tests, including measurement of inspiratory and expiratory pressure as well as a forced tidal volume, might be helpful.[14–16] Patients with severe diaphragmatic weakness have a decreased vital capacity that is usually less than 1 L (normal: 40–70 mL/kg or 3–5 L). The maximal inspiratory pressure and the maximal expiratory pressure are around ~ 80 cm of H_2O under normal conditions. These pressures become clearly insufficient to create inward airflow if they reach the 30–40 cm H_2O range.[17–19]

Obviously, it is important to seek additional contributing factors such as aspiration or ongoing pneumonia that can be demonstrated on a routine chest X-ray. The most commonly asked question for neurologists is, "does this patient have a respiratory failure of neuromuscular origin?" and "should the underlying neurologic disorder be emergently treated?"

Myasthenia gravis may present with eyelid drooping, episodic double vision (sometimes inadvertently leading to inappropriate corrective surgery), and, in more severe cases, generalized fatigue and weakness. Patients with myasthenia gravis may develop a "crisis," which is often simply defined as the presence of respiratory failure but can be better understood as a rapidly evolving, life-threatening respiratory failure and inability to clear secretions causing double trouble. Neuromuscular respiratory failure in myasthenia gravis (but also in other causes) is associated with increased breathing effort. When this effort is profound, patients appear clinically restless, anxious, and uncomfortable and may have clamminess and sweating on the forehead. Options for respiratory support include noninvasive ventilation with bilevel positive airway pressure (BiPAP), and endotracheal intubation and mechanical ventilation. Treatment for myasthenia gravis involves corticosteroids, plasma exchange or intravenous immunoglobulin (IVIG), and pyridostigmine. Plasma exchange may involve five to seven exchanges of 2–3 L each, usually every other day. Timely diagnosis and appropriate treatment for patients with bulbar and respiratory muscle weakness have reduced the seriousness of the clinical course and time of hospital stay. However, elderly patients with a myasthenic crisis complicated by aspiration pneumonia may have a prolonged hospital stay even with early recognition and treatment.

THE PRESENTING CLINICAL PROBLEM

In this simulation, a 60-year-old female presents with shortness of breath, recent fever, blurred vision for the last 24 h, and repeated coughing. Over the past several days, she has had flu-like symptoms. The learning objectives are to take a proper history and recognize diplopia, dysphagia, change in voice, and worsening with fatigue or time of day, sleeping position, and difficulty with climbing stairs, combing hair, or brushing teeth. The learner should recognize the patient might have myasthenia gravis and perform a focused neuromuscular examination with attention to fatigability. In addition, the learner should get a chest X-ray and arterial blood gas as well as other appropriate laboratory studies that would narrow the differential of acute weakness. The learner should recognize the need for assisted ventilation and initiate medical management. The learner should also discuss the need for IVIG or PLEX and consider the appropriateness of pyridostigmine. In addition, the learner should consider the need, safety, and dosing of corticosteroids. The main objectives are listed in Table 11.1 and key competencies are shown in Fig. 11.1.

Preparation

The additional equipment and scenario setup are detailed in Table 11.2. The patient is sitting up, leaning

---

TABLE 11.1
Objectives

- Recognize subtle signs of neuromuscular respiratory failure
- Diagnose myasthenia gravis based on history and examination
- Interpret pulmonary function tests, arterial blood gas, and chest X-ray
- Assess need for mechanical ventilation
- Provide appropriate noninvasive assisted ventilation
- Develop an appropriate treatment plan

---

forward, in bed in the emergency department. The monitor shows a blood pressure of 160/90 mmHg; heart rate of 113 beats/min; and respiratory rate of 33 per minute. The oxygen saturation is 95% on 2 L of oxygen via nasal cannula. The patient has a few drops of sweat on the forehead.

Coaching Actors

The actor is specifically asked not to volunteer information unless asked. This will allow the learner to come gradually to the complete history and diagnosis. The actor is coached to speak with short truncated sentences and to pause frequently. The actor should take a breath in the middle of each sentence. The actor is instructed to shrug shoulders slightly with each inspiration to mimic sternocleidomastoid muscle use. If the patient is put in a supine position, the respiration should speed up a bit, and the actor can say she is uncomfortable and get back up. With some training, it is possible to act out a very believable shortness of breath as a result of mechanical respiratory weakness. Many actors are perfectly able to demonstrate abdominal paradox by moving the abdomen in with every inspiration to reduce chest expansion. Generally, the actor may display some degree of anxiety and restlessness as is commonly seen in nearly decompensating patients (Table 11.3). Fatigable strength may be portrayed as initially strong but, with second testing and third testing, may show a progressive give way. In our experience, learners may recognize that this progressive give way represents fatigable weakness or at least that weakness is present. (Learners—when properly prebriefed—will understand we are not simulating functional weakness). Some actors are even able to imitate a "myasthenic snarl" indicative of bifacial palsy.

THE IDEAL LEARNER

L introduces himself and proceeds to inquire about the patient's symptoms. *P* will tell him that she has been feeling ill for a week or so, and today she is unable to swallow her cough medication. *P* will also tell *L* that she has had blurred vision continuously over the last 24 h. *L* asks what is meant by blurred vision and if anything makes it better or worse and is told that it usually occurs when she is very fatigued and that it gets better when she closes one eye. *L* leads *P* through a focused neuromuscular review of systems and learns that *P* has found it harder to climb stairs or comb her hair, she feels that her voice is softer than normal, and she has been sleeping most of the night in a chair.

All these cues should point to the possible diagnosis of myasthenia gravis. *L* then performs a basic examination focused on detecting myasthenia gravis. This includes looking upward at the learner's finger. When *P* complains of seeing double, *L* recognizes progressive ptosis. On testing, neck, arm, or leg strength should be initially strong, but rechecking the same muscles reveals weakness. Biting on a tongue depressor, *P* is easily able to initially resist any attempt to pull it away but on repeat testing cannot do so. *P* is unable to count to 10 in one breath. *L* asks *P* to lie flat to test for paradoxical breathing and recognizes it immediately.[20] *L* concludes that *P* has a neuromuscular respiratory failure and considers myasthenia gravis as the main cause. *L* requests an arterial blood gas, chest X-ray, and pulmonary function tests (Table 11.4). *CONF* asks, "Do you think the patient needs intubation?" *L* reviews the requested tests, noting bibasilar atelectasis, low vital capacity, maximal expiratory and inspiratory pressures, and an unexpectedly normal pCO_2 despite hyperventilation (suggesting early respiratory failure) and recommends initiation of BiPAP, clearly and effectively discussing this with the patient. When BiPAP has been started, *L* triages *P* to the intensive care unit.[14,21–23] *L* orders IVIG or PLEX treatment, low-dose pyridostigmine, and 10 mg of prednisone. He then discusses the possible need for endotracheal intubation with *P*. Scenario ends.

THE NOT-SO IDEAL LEARNER

1. *The learner does not make the appropriate diagnosis.* The most common mistake is to not recognize that the patient has fatigable weakness and that respiratory failure worsens when changing the patient to a supine position. Many learners do recognize the staccato-type speech, change in voice, and frontal sweat as signs of respiratory failure, and some may pursue other respiratory causes such as a pulmonary

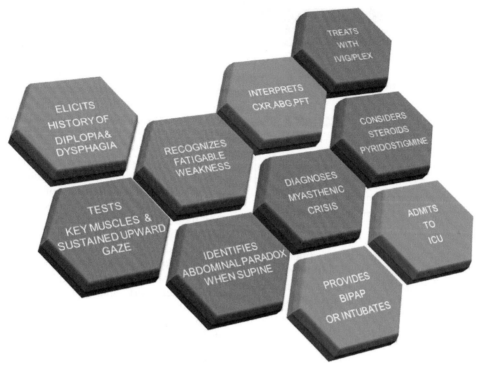

FIG. 11.1 Deconstructing key competencies in acute neuromuscular respiratory failure.

TABLE 11.2 Scenario Setup for Neuromuscular Respiratory Failure	
People Needed	• Actor to play the patient • Actor to play the emergency department nurse • Attending or NCC fellow to facilitate
Equipment needed	• Laboratory results • Syringes • Blood pressure cuff • IV line • Reflex hammer • Oxygen by nasal cannula • BiPAP mask
Setup needed	• IV line • Blood pressure cuff on actor • Monitor setup from various sources • Monitor showing sinus rhythm, elevated blood pressure, and chest X-ray

TABLE 11.3 Actor Instructions Before Simulation
• Complain of blurry vision (if asked what is meant by blurry state "I see two of everything")
• Practice developing ptosis on sustained upward gaze
• Mildly increased respiratory rate
• Pause after every 4 or 5 words
• Gradually display a worsening respiratory rate and complain of shortness of breath
• Complain of shortness of breath when lying down and move the abdomen in with inspiration
• Try to shrug shoulders slightly when breathing in
• Show fatigable weakness
• May volunteer difficulty with swallowing

TABLE 11.4
Tests in Acute Neuromuscular Respiratory Failure

Test	Findings	Comments
Chest X-ray	• Elevated hemidiaphragm • Infiltrates • Atelectasis	• May be preexisting • May indicate aspiration or prior infection • Indicate low tidal volumes
Arterial blood gas	• Hypercarbia • Normal $PaCO_2$ with tachypnea • Normal	• Late finding • Early failing • Common finding
Pulmonary function test	• Reduced (<30%) vital capacity • Maximal inspiratory and expiratory pressures	• Effort is important • Leakage from bifacial palsy may be overcome with mask spirometry
EMG	• Reduced CMAP amplitude • Phrenic nerve, fibrillation potentials • Short-duration MUP	• No clear benefit in acute setting
Ultrasound diaphragm	• Reduced diaphragm excursion	• May have benefit in acute setting

CMAP, compound muscle action potential; *MUP*, motor unit potential; *PaCO₂*: Partial pressure of carbon dioxide in arterial blood.

embolus when no explanation is found on chest X-ray. Most learners will expect to see a neurologic disorder when going through a simulation course such as this and will eventually come to some presumptive diagnosis.

2. *The learner does not recognize a subtle abnormality in blood gas and pulmonary function testing.* Many learners focus on the blood gas value, which appears normal, but are unaware that patients with neuromuscular respiratory failure initially have normal blood gases and that the normal $PaCO_2$ is, in fact, abnormal in the context of hyperventilation. Indeed, one would expect a lower $PaCO_2$, but the diaphragm cannot provide adequate ventilation.

3. *The learner does not recognize that BiPAP is beneficial.* Once the patient is recognized as being in respiratory failure, learners often fail to conclude that the patient would benefit from noninvasive mechanical ventilation, which, in many cases, prevents the need for endotracheal intubation.

4. *The learner does not consider IVIG or plasma exchange.* We expect most physicians to be aware of immunotherapy or plasma exchange to treat myasthenia gravis particularly when they present in a crisis and increasing doses of pyridostigmine have resulted in more secretions.

5. *The learner does not triage to an ICU.* Triage to a neurointensive care unit or any other intensive care unit or at least a monitored bed will be needed for close monitoring.

ADAPTING THE SCENARIO

The level of difficulty can be adjusted to the learner's needs. If the learner is unable to diagnose myasthenia gravis, the facilitator may elect to provide the diagnosis and then have the learner do the appropriate tests. It is often more important to recognize neuromuscular respiratory failure rather than the underlying cause. The scenario can be adapted for different learners with different objectives. For example, neurology residents should recognize myasthenia gravis while an emergency medicine resident should recognize that the patient might benefit from noninvasive mechanical ventilation. The severity of respiratory failure can be adjusted (moulage to create sweat on the forehead) and episodic hypoxemia (adjusted by the instructor behind the mirror). For any learner, it will be important to fully understand the risks of wrong triage and delayed treatment.

DEBRIEFING

Discussion of the main principles of mechanical respiratory failure will be reviewed. The session should emphasize the subtleties of diaphragmatic failure such as (1) mild tachycardia and tachypnea and having to sit upright, (2) frequently halting speech as a result of poor mechanics, and (3) perspiration on the forehead.

The debriefing can be used to discuss appropriate initial treatment of myasthenic crisis and how to decide between the various options. It can also touch on indications for intubation versus noninvasive mechanical ventilation and their relationship to secretion management and initiation of corticosteroids and their inherent risk of transient worsening of the myasthenic symptoms. The debriefing session will emphasize the key competencies, why decisions were good, and which were problematic. Additional videos on the respiratory mechanics of established patients can be shown to emphasize the staccato speech and paradoxical breathing. Tests that can be helpful in assessing acute neuromuscular failure are shown in Table 11.4 can be discussed in more detail during the debriefing session.

CONCLUSIONS

Simulating neuromuscular respiratory failure is feasible in the simulation center. Our actors are able to mimic shortness of breath, halting speech, and provide clues to the diagnosis by telling the learner about their diplopia and dysphagia when they appear to be off track. In our experience, we have been able adequately to simulate myasthenia gravis causing respiratory failure. Few props are necessary to provide an ideal teaching situation.

REFERENCES

1. Alshekhlee A, Miles JD, Katirji B, et al. Incidence and mortality rates of myasthenia gravis and myasthenic crisis in US hospitals. *Neurology.* 2009;72:1548–1554.
2. Thomas CE, Mayer SA, Gungor Y, et al. Myasthenic crisis: clinical features, mortality, complications, and risk factors for prolonged intubation. *Neurology.* 1997;48:1253–1260.
3. Cabrera Serrano M, Rabinstein AA. Causes and outcomes of acute neuromuscular respiratory failure. *Arch Neurol.* 2010;67:1089–1094.
4. Bolton CF, Chen R, Wijdicks EFM, et al. *Neurology of Breathing.* Amsterdam: Elsevier; 2004.
5. Burakgazi AZ, Hoke A. Respiratory muscle weakness in peripheral neuropathies. *J Peripher Nerv Syst.* 2010;15: 307–313.
6. Derenne JP, Macklem PT, Roussos C. The respiratory muscles: mechanics, control, and pathophysiology. *Am Rev Respir Dis.* 1978;118:119–133.
7. Derenne JP, Macklem PT, Roussos C. The respiratory muscles: mechanics, control, and pathophysiology. *Part 2 Am Rev Respir Dis.* 1978;118:373–390.
8. Derenne JP, Macklem PT, Roussos C. The respiratory muscles: mechanics, control, and pathophysiology. *Part III. Am Rev Respir Dis.* 1978;118:581–601.
9. Guyenet PG, Bayliss DA. Neural control of breathing and CO2 homeostasis. *Neuron.* 2015;87:946–961.
10. Hughes RA, Bihari D. Acute neuromuscular respiratory paralysis. *J Neurol Neurosurg Psychiatry.* 1993;56:334–343.
11. Laghi F, Tobin MJ. Disorders of the respiratory muscles. *Am J Respir Crit Care Med.* 2003;168:10–48.
12. Wijdicks EFM. The neurology of acutely failing respiratory mechanics. *Ann Neurol.* 2017;81:485–494.
13. Galtrey CM, Faulkner M, Wren DR. How it feels to experience three different causes of respiratory failure. *Pract Neurol.* 2012;12:49–54.
14. Lawn ND, Fletcher DD, Henderson RD, et al. Anticipating mechanical ventilation in Guillain-Barre syndrome. *Arch Neurol.* 2001;58:893–898.
15. Sharshar T, Chevret S, Bourdain F, et al. Early predictors of mechanical ventilation in Guillain-Barre syndrome. *Crit Care Med.* 2003;31:278–283.
16. Walgaard C, Lingsma HF, Ruts L, et al. Prediction of respiratory insufficiency in Guillain-Barre syndrome. *Ann Neurol.* 2010;67:781–787.
17. Cohen CA, Zagelbaum G, Gross D, et al. Clinical manifestations of inspiratory muscle fatigue. *Am J Med.* 1982;73: 308–316.
18. Kramer CL, McCullough M, Wijdicks EF. Teaching video neuroimages: how to unmask respiratory strength confounded by facial diplegia. *Neurology.* 2015;84:e57–58.
19. Walterspacher S, Kirchberger A, Lambeck J, et al. Respiratory muscle assessment in acute Guillain-Barre syndrome. *Lung.* 2016;194:821–828.
20. Fromageot C, Lofaso F, Annane D, et al. Supine fall in lung volumes in the assessment of diaphragmatic weakness in neuromuscular disorders. *Arch Phys Med Rehabil.* 2001; 82:123–128.
21. Frat JP, Thille AW, Mercat A, et al. High-flow oxygen through nasal cannula in acute hypoxemic respiratory failure. *N Engl J Med.* 2015;372:2185–2196.
22. Mehta S, Hill NS. Noninvasive ventilation. *Am J Respir Crit Care Med.* 2001;163:540–577.
23. Hess DR. Noninvasive ventilation for neuromuscular disease. *Clin Chest Med.* 2018;39:437–447.

CHAPTER 12

Simulating Status Epilepticus

Status epilepticus (SE) is a complex condition most commonly first encountered in the emergency department, but all hospitalists and intensivists should be trained in its management. The hard truth is that few are. Seizures evolving into status epilepticus often overwhelm fellows rotating on rapid-response teams, and triage to an ICU may occur without appropriate first-line treatment. Some seizures are clear pseudoseizures or other movement disorders such as myoclonus, and many are treated with inadequate doses of benzodiazepine out of concern for airway compromise, leading to ongoing seizures and resultant respiratory compromise and ICU admission. Moreover, the differential diagnosis is broad and includes all acute encephalopathies, drug or alcohol intoxication and withdrawal, and central nervous system infections. In truth, this is a major neuroemergency.

Expert management of SE requires physicians simultaneously to (1) diagnose the disorder early, (2) stop the seizures, (3) search for their cause and initiate treatment when available, and (4) anticipate and treat systemic complications. In our simulation center, we have developed a scenario that uses well-trained actors rather than a mannequin programmed to display the not-so-realistic herky-jerky movements that are supposed to represent "convulsions." Actors can adequately mimic a seizure and enable us to simulate a number of major decision points.

THE PROBLEM BEFORE US

Status epilepticus occurs infrequently in adults, but every ICU can count on at least three to four admissions per month. SE is a condition of self-sustaining seizures resulting from either failure of inhibitory mechanisms responsible for seizure termination or from ongoing activation of excitatory mechanisms.[1] Specifically, synaptic GABA$_A$ and glutamate receptors are trafficked off the membrane or internalized, causing failure of GABAergic inhibition and an increase in glutamatergic excitation. AMPA- and NMDA-receptor subunits move to the synaptic membrane, where they form additional excitatory receptors.[2-7] This change in receptors may influence which antiseizure drugs to use—GABA agonists

(i.e., benzodiazepines) first and NMDA inhibitors (i.e., ketamine) later. SE can have long-term consequences, including neuronal injury and epileptogenesis, depending on the type and duration of SE.[2,8-15]

Patients may manifest overt convulsions or, to the newcomer, show no recognizable clinical signs at all depending on the seizure type, location, extent of cortex involved, and the duration of seizures.[1,16,17] The recognition of dyscognitive focal (previously called complex partial) SE can be particularly difficult because it starts gradually in most cases with an aura before evolving to produce impairment of cognitive function with overt confusion or impaired consciousness. This type of SE can be mistaken for acute stroke as patients may be mute and staring into space. The presence of repetitive automatisms (performance of actions without conscious thought or intention or small-amplitude twitching movements of the face, hands, or feet) provides clues to the diagnosis. Frontal epileptic foci can produce bizarre behaviors, and patients have been inaccurately diagnosed with a psychotic break.

Treatment of status epilepticus is not well settled. Frequent treatment algorithm adjustments often occur on the basis of personal preference and nothing more. What all epileptologists and neurointensivists agree on is that the initial treatment of choice is a benzodiazepine.[18] Benzodiazepines are inadequately used but, when prescribed in accordance with guidelines, improve seizure control and patient outcomes.[19,20] Furthermore, underdosing of benzodiazepines and consequent continued seizure activity are more likely to lead to airway complications and hypoxemic respiratory failure than adequate benzodiazepine administration.[21,22] Consensus exists that all patients should be treated immediately with a second antiseizure drug to prevent seizure recurrence even when benzodiazepines abort seizures. An ongoing, randomized, controlled trial compares fosphenytoin, levetiracetam, and valproate at maximum doses for benzodiazepine refractory SE.[23] Currently, all three of these drugs are supported by guidelines along with phenobarbital.[24,25] Recent experience also suggests that polytherapy, in particular with a

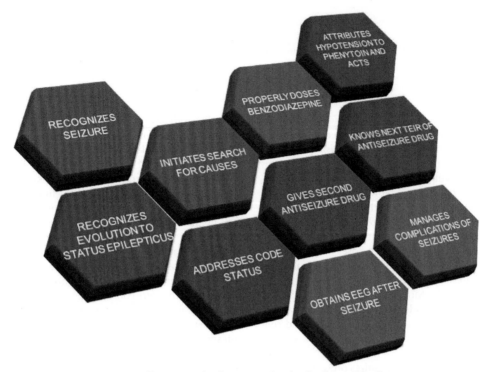

FIG. 12.1 Deconstructing key competencies in status epilepticus.

combination of low-dose midazolam, ketamine, and valproate, may perform better both in cessation of SE and reduction of posttreatment seizures.[26] Options for third-line therapy include continuous infusion of intravenous (IV) anesthetic drugs (favored in generalized convulsive SE) and all fast-acting IV, nonanesthetic antiseizure drugs.

EEG is necessary to exclude ongoing electrographic seizures after cessation of clinical manifestations if the patient does not recover to baseline within 10 min, as nonconvulsive seizures are seen on continuous EEG monitoring in 48% of adults and up to 57% of children following convulsive seizures.[24,27,28] EEG thus becomes a tool that monitors the adequacy of treatment. Etiology is the primary determinant of outcome;[17,29,30] thus, rapid recognition and treatment of the cause of SE may impact patient outcome if treatment other than seizure control is needed (e.g., autoimmune encephalitis).

SE results in a host of acute systemic (predominantly cardiopulmonary) complications. Respiratory failure, associated with poor outcome, occurs in one-third of SE episodes as a result of apnea, mucous plugging causing upper-airway obstruction, neurocardiogenic pulmonary edema, or aspiration of gastric contents.[31] Cardiac arrest in status epilepticus is very uncommon

(approximately 1%) but may be related to cause of status epilepticus (drug-related), hypoxemia, prior comorbidity, or direct cardiac injury.[32] Two-thirds of patients have markers of cardiac injury including electrocardiogram changes, troponin elevation, and cardiac arrhythmias, the presence of which is associated with poor outcomes.[33] In addition to cardiopulmonary complications, patients can develop rhabdomyolysis, renal failure, musculoskeletal mechanical injuries, and rarely disseminated intravascular coagulation. This multifaceted medical emergency allows for many approaches to simulation of status epilepticus. The key components of simulating status epilepticus and its initial management are shown in Fig. 12.1; the objectives are shown in Table 12.1.

THE PRESENTING CLINICAL PROBLEM

The patient is a 68-year-old right-handed man with hypertension, hyperlipidemia, and a prior stroke 3 years ago presenting with "confusion" and left-sided weakness.

The learner must differentiate focal dyscognitive SE (mute, staring, fidgeting) from acute ischemic stroke and other mimicking conditions and then appropriately manage the situation as it evolves into convulsive SE. While the scenario can be easily adapted for different

TABLE 12.1
Objectives

- Recognize seizure
- Direct appropriate pharmacologic treatment
- Escalate antiseizure drugs step-by-step
- Consider cause of status epilepticus
- Manage complications of seizures
- Know the side effects of antiseizure drugs

learners, the patient in our scenario has new-onset focal epilepsy due to a remote ischemic stroke (clue provided by the patient's spouse, who describes a "transient ischemic attack"). Our scenario also includes changing a do-not-intubate status for a treatable disorder.

Preparation

The patient lies in a hospital bed in the ED with a peripheral intravenous catheter inserted and vital signs showing on the monitor. Two weeks before the simulation, learners receive status epilepticus guidelines to review in advance of the training.[24,25] Additional setup and equipment required are detailed in Table 12.2.

Coaching Actors

Detailed instructions are shown in Table 12.3. The actor begins the scenario with eyes open and looking forward. He is hemiparetic on the left. He does not make eye contact with anyone (as though he is in his own world). He fidgets with his right hand and spontaneously moves his right leg. When tapped on the foot (by the nurse), he has a brief, generalized seizure. Whenever he receives a foot-tap signal, he begins another convulsive seizure. His eyes remain open during the seizure (see Chapter 2, Fig. 2.4B).

The primary role of the patient's spouse is to field questions about the history of present illness, medical history, and code status. She receives coaching to appear appropriately worried and answers the learner's questions according to the script provided. When the convulsive seizures first begin, the spouse reacts with surprise and asks, "What is happening to him?" The spouse also introduces a communication challenge for the learner with respect to code status. If the learner or the nurse mentions "intubation" aloud (or if the learner asks the spouse directly), the spouse indicates that her husband does not want to be intubated and that he has been very clear about his preferences in this regard.

Indent if at any point the learner seems lost, the facilitator can prompt the nurse to ask probing questions such as "What do you think is going on?" or "What does the CT scan show?" to redirect.

THE IDEAL LEARNER

L introduces herself to the patient, spouse, and nurse (*CONF*). She then quickly observes that the patient is awake but not responsive and notes that he moves his right side spontaneously but does not move the left side. L proceeds to take a focused history from P's spouse. She is careful to clarify that the changes began somewhat gradually rather than suddenly. L requests a noncontrast head CT scan and laboratory studies.

L then states she is going to examine P and directs her attention to the patient. Upon examination, she finds the patient awake but inattentive. He is not fixating or tracking at all. He blinks to threat bilaterally. He is mute and does not follow commands. She notes that he picks repetitively at his shirt with the right hand and that this can be interrupted briefly.

L reviews the laboratory results and notes they are normal except for the lactate, creatine kinase, glucose, and white blood cell count, which are moderately elevated, and the serum bicarbonate, which is low. She then reviews the CT scan, which is normal, specifically noting the absence of hemorrhage, hypodensity, extraaxial fluid collection, hydrocephalus, or hyperdense MCA sign. Just as L finishes reviewing the CT scan, *CONF* taps P's foot, and he has a generalized convulsive seizure. L turns to note the seizure and vital signs changes showing BP 190/101 mmHg, pulse 132 beats/min, and oxygen saturation 92%. L inquires about IV access and is told there are two peripheral IVs in place. She instructs the nurse to give 4 mg IV lorazepam now thinking he may have been in focal dyscognitive SE all along and orders 20 mg/kg IV fosphenytoin to be given at a rate of 150 mg/min. P stops convulsing. He lies in bed with eyes closed and extremities flaccid. L orders an emergent EEG to exclude ongoing nonconvulsive seizures. *CONF* taps P's foot to begin another convulsive seizure. L instructs the nurse to give another 4 mg IV lorazepam. She observes the patient and notes he has an oxygen saturation of 88%. While elevated during the prior convulsive seizure, BP is now 90/50 mmHg and pulse is 60 beats/min. She tells *CONF* to start oxygen by nasal cannula, to hold the fosphenytoin infusion temporarily, and to give a liter of normal saline. L then anticipates possible intubation.

TABLE 12.2
Scenario Setup for Status Epilepticus

People needed	• Actor to play the patient • Actor to play the nurse • Actor to portray patient's spouse • Attending or NCC fellow to facilitate
Equipment needed	• Monitor display: • Blood pressure 125/50 mmHg • Pulse 65 • SpO₂ 96% room air • Respiratory rate 16 • Temp 38.0°C
Setup needed	• Electrocardiogram • CT scan • Flashlight • IV lorazepam, IM and IV midazolam, bags of fosphenytoin, levetiracetam, valproate sodium and phenobarbital • IV access • Intubation kit
Preparation	• Patient lying in hospital bed with IV catheters inserted and blood pressure cuff/telemetry leads attached

SpO2, peripheral capillary oxygen saturation; *IV*, intravenous; *ED*, emergency department; *CT*, computed tomography.

TABLE 12.3
Instructions for Actor Before Simulation

• Do not make eye contact with anyone

• Fidget with right hand (pick at shirt or roll fingers together)

• Portray seizure as flexing arms, extending neck and legs.

• Roll eyes up or sideways

• Keep eyelids open during seizure and closed in between seizures

• Seizure duration: ∼30 seconds

L (turning to spouse): "We may need to insert a tube temporarily to help him breathe. This would just be until the seizures are controlled and he wakes up enough to protect his airway."

L turns to *P* and sees that the blood pressure and pulse have normalized, oxygen saturation is 85% on 4-L nasal cannula, and the patient remains unresponsive. Noting the low-grade fever, she orders blood cultures and empiric treatment with acyclovir, ceftriaxone, and vancomycin for possible meningoencephalitis.

CONF hands the EEG to *L* (Fig. 12.2 top), and *L* says "this shows generalized spike and waves suggesting that he is still seizing." *L* asks *CONF* to give 3 more mg of IV lorazepam (total 0.1 mg/kg), resume the fosphenytoin infusion at 100 mg/min, and prepare to intubate *P*.

CONF leaves an endotracheal tube on the pillow to provide a visual reminder that the airway is secured and says "the patient is now intubated." *L* requests urgent admission to the neurointensive care unit, where the patient can undergo spinal fluid examination and continuous EEG monitoring until he wakes up. *CONF* hands a new EEG to *L* (Fig. 12.2 bottom). *L* explains to *P*'s spouse that the seizures have now stopped. Scenario ends.

THE NOT-SO-IDEAL LEARNER

We have identified the following common missteps:

1. The learner anchors on the diagnosis of stroke. If the learner does not elicit the correct history, fixes on stroke, and initiates acute stroke care, the nurse will cue the actor to start a convulsive seizure to clarify the situation.

2. The learner hesitates and does not take charge. Learner takes a very long, thorough history (because she is unsure of how to proceed). Again, a cue to the actor to begin a seizure should prompt the learner to action.

3. The learner undertreats or waits too long to treat seizures. She does not give additional benzodiazepine after oxygen saturation drops (so seizures continue) or fails to give a second antiseizure drug after benzodiazepine. The scenario ends if there is no step-by-step escalation of antiseizure drugs.

4. The learner devotes insufficient attention to the "ABCs" (airway, breathing, and circulation). She does not address the hypoxemia or over-reacts. She does not treat the hypotension because it was "not that low." She does not attribute the hypotension to the fosphenytoin and, as a result, does not pause the infusion or provide fluids. Consequently, the hypotension gets worse and leads to pulseless electrical activity. Here the scenario ends.

5. The learner communicates poorly with the patient's spouse. She ignores her or fails to provide any reassurance. The part of the scenario that deals with escalation of drugs and thus temporary intubation remains important and should be handled well.

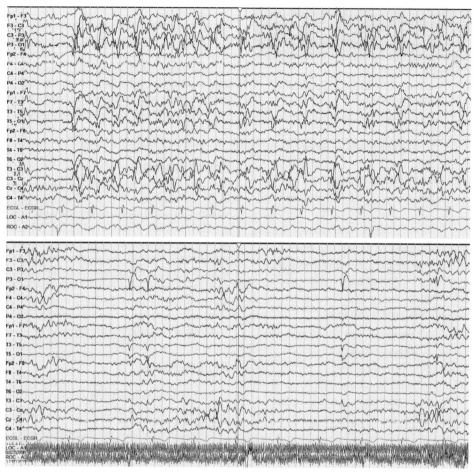

FIG. 12.2 Electroencephalogram provided before (top) and after (bottom) treatment.

ADAPTING THE SCENARIO

The difficulty level is adjusted to the learner's needs. If the learner is struggling, the facilitator may elect not to add additional pitfalls to the management but rather to end the scenario and cover the remaining competencies in the post-scenario debrief.

This scenario can also be easily adapted for learners with differing objectives. For example, the diagnosis may be made less challenging for learners with less neurologic background by removing the hemiparesis, or by having paramedics, or family provide history of a witnessed seizure at home, allowing more time to focus on evaluation and treatment. Because our scenario primarily targets neurology residents, we make

the diagnosis challenging to force consideration of a broader differential diagnosis. For learners in critical care, the focus may shift to seizure management and timing of intubation. Other competencies that can be incorporated into adaptations of this scenario include recognition and management of systemic complications. The patient could desaturate to test the learner's clinical judgment with respect to airway management. If intravenous fosphenytoin is administered, the patient may develop a tachyarrhythmia such as ventricular tachycardia. We tend to focus on status epilepticus management but systemic complications—particularly management of cardiogenic shock from stress cardiomyopathy—can be built into the scenario.

TABLE 12.4
Pharmacologic Options for the Treatment of Status Epilepticus in 3 Stages

EARLY (FIRST-LINE THERAPY)	
Lorazepam	0.1 mg/kg IV up to 4 mg per dose, may repeat in 5 min
Diazepam	0.15 mg/kg IV up to 10 mg per dose, may repeat in 5 min
Midazolam	0.2 mg/kg IM up to maximum of 10 mg
ESTABLISHED (SECOND-LINE THERAPY)	
Valproate sodium	20–40 mg/kg IV; 3–6 mg/kg/min
Fosphenytoin	20 mg PE/kg IV; up to 150 mg PE/min
Phenytoin	20 mg/kg IV; up to 50 mg/min
Phenobarbital	20 mg/kg IV; 50–100 mg/min, may give in 10 mg/kg increments
Levetiracetam	20–60 mg/kg IV; 2–5 mg/kg/min
REFRACTORY (THIRD-LINE THERAPY)	
Midazolam	0.2 mg/kg LD, then 0.05–2 mg/kg/hr
Propofol*	1–2 mg/kg LD, then 30–200 mcg/kg/min
Pentobarbital	5–15 mg/kg LD, then 0.5–5 mg/kg/h
Thiopental	2–7 mg/kg LD, then 0.5–5 mg/kg/h
Valproate sodium	See above
Levetiracetam	See above
Phenobarbital	See above
Phenytoin/ fosphenytoin	See above
Lacosamide	200–400 mg IV, then 100–200 mg IV twice daily
Topiramate	200–400 mg NG/PO, then 300–1600 mg/day (divided two to four times daily)

IV, intravenous; *NG*, nasogastric; *PO*, per os (by mouth).
*Caution risk of propofol infusion syndrome at doses >80 mcg/kg/min for >14 h.
see Iyer VN, Hoel R, Rabinstein AA. Propofol infusion syndrome in patients with refractory status epilepticus: an 11-year clinical experience. *Crit Care Med*. 2009;37:3024–3030.

DEBRIEFING

Particular attention is paid to developing the differential diagnosis, proper pharmacologic treatment of status epilepticus, airway management, and evaluation of the cause of new-onset seizures. Evidence is reviewed for the pharmacologic treatment of SE, and pitfalls and the advantages of each drug are discussed. The options for treatment of status epilepticus are shown in Table 12.4. Debriefing can focus on maximizing the dose of benzodiazepines, rapid administration of a second-line antiseizure drug, and the cardiovascular effects of phenytoin and fosphenytoin. Timing of EEG, investigation into the cause of SE, indications for lumbar puncture, and screening for systemic complications are all reviewed.

CONCLUSIONS

A number of important decision points can be identified, and the essentials of adequate management of seizures or status epilepticus can be simulated. For learners, it is important to get a better handle on step-by-step escalation of IV drugs and recognition of major side effects. Algorithms on management of status epilepticus change frequently, and the correct sequence and doses may not be known. For the learner, it is most important to know how to support the patient, treat seizures successfully, know the pharmacopeia, and initiate a search for the cause.

REFERENCES

1. Trinka E, Cock H, Hesdorffer D, et al. A definition and classification of status epilepticus—report of the ILAE Task Force on Classification of Status Epilepticus. *Epilepsia*. 2015;56:1515–1523.
2. Meldrum BS, Horton RW. Physiology of status epilepticus in primates. *Arch Neurol*. 1973;28:1–9.
3. Kapur J, Macdonald RL. Rapid seizure-induced reduction of benzodiazepine and Zn2+ sensitivity of hippocampal dentate granule cell GABAA receptors. *J Neurosci*. 1997; 17:7532–7540.
4. Naylor DE, Liu H, Wasterlain CG. Trafficking of GABA(A) receptors, loss of inhibition, and a mechanism for pharmacoresistance in status epilepticus. *J Neurosci*. 2005;25: 7724–7733.
5. Goodkin HP, Sun C, Yeh JL, et al. GABA(A) receptor internalization during seizures. *Epilepsia*. 2007;48(suppl 5): 109–113.
6. Niquet J, Baldwin R, Suchomelova L, et al. Benzodiazepine-refractory status epilepticus: pathophysiology and principles of treatment. *Ann N Y Acad Sci*. 2016;1378:166–173.
7. Naylor DE, Liu H, Niquet J, et al. Rapid surface accumulation of NMDA receptors increases glutamatergic excitation during status epilepticus. *Neurobiol Dis*. 2013;54:225–238.
8. Elliott RC, Miles MF, Lowenstein DH. Overlapping microarray profiles of dentate gyrus gene expression during development- and epilepsy-associated neurogenesis and axon outgrowth. *J Neurosci*. 2003;23:2218–2227.
9. Roopra A, Dingledine R, Hsieh J. Epigenetics and epilepsy. *Epilepsia*. 2012;53(suppl 9):2–10.

10. Jimenez-Mateos EM, Henshall DC. Epilepsy and microRNA. *Neuroscience.* 2013;238:218−229.
11. Meldrum BS, Vigouroux RA, Brierley JB. Systemic factors and epileptic brain damage. Prolonged seizures in paralyzed, artificially ventilated baboons. *Arch Neurol.* 1973; 29:82−87.
12. Sloviter RS. Decreased hippocampal inhibition and a selective loss of interneurons in experimental epilepsy. *Science.* 1987;235:73−76.
13. Sankar R, Shin DH, Liu H, et al. Patterns of status epilepticus-induced neuronal injury during development and long-term consequences. *J Neurosci.* 1998;18: 8382−8393.
14. Chuang YC, Chang AY, Lin JW, et al. Mitochondrial dysfunction and ultrastructural damage in the hippocampus during kainic acid-induced status epilepticus in the rat. *Epilepsia.* 2004;45:1202−1209.
15. Lopez-Meraz ML, Niquet J, Wasterlain CG. Distinct caspase pathways mediate necrosis and apoptosis in subpopulations of hippocampal neurons after status epilepticus. *Epilepsia.* 2010;51(suppl 3):56−60.
16. Meierkord H, Holtkamp M. Non-convulsive status epilepticus in adults: clinical forms and treatment. *Lancet Neurol.* 2007;6:329−339.
17. Lowenstein DH, Alldredge BK. Status epilepticus. *N Engl J Med.* 1998;338:970−976.
18. Treiman DM, Meyers PD, Walton NY, et al. A comparison of four treatments for generalized convulsive status epilepticus. Veterans Affairs Status Epilepticus Cooperative Study Group. *N Engl J Med.* 1998;339:792−798.
19. Braun J, Gau E, Revelle S, et al. Impact of non-guideline-based treatment of status epilepticus. *J Neurol Sci.* 2017; 382:126−130.
20. Aranda A, Foucart G, Ducasse JL, et al. Generalized convulsive status epilepticus management in adults: a cohort study with evaluation of professional practice. *Epilepsia.* 2010;51:2159−2167.
21. Chamberlain JM, Altieri MA, Futterman C, et al. A prospective, randomized study comparing intramuscular midazolam with intravenous diazepam for the treatment of seizures in children. *Pediatr Emerg Care.* 1997;13: 92−94.
22. Silbergleit R, Biros MH, Harney D, et al. Implementation of the exception from informed consent regulations in a large multicenter emergency clinical trials network: the RAMPART experience. *Acad Emerg Med.* 2012;19: 448−454.
23. Cock HR, Group E. Established status epilepticus treatment trial (ESETT). *Epilepsia.* 2011;52(suppl 8):50−52.
24. Brophy GM, Bell R, Claassen J, et al. Guidelines for the evaluation and management of status epilepticus. *Neurocrit Care.* 2012;17:3−23.
25. Glauser T, Shinnar S, Gloss D, et al. Evidence-based guideline: treatment of convulsive status epilepticus in children and adults: report of the guideline committee of the American epilepsy Society. *Epilepsy Curr.* 2016;16:48−61.
26. Niquet J, Baldwin R, Norman K, et al. Drug combinations targeting GABA and glutamate networks in the treatment of status epilepticus. In: American Epilepsy Society Annual Meeting 2017. Washington DC.
27. Claassen J, Taccone FS, Horn P, et al. Recommendations on the use of EEG monitoring in critically ill patients: consensus statement from the neurointensive care section of the ESICM. *Intensive Care Med.* 2013;39:1337−1351.
28. Herman ST, Abend NS, Bleck TP, et al. Consensus statement on continuous EEG in critically ill adults and children, part I: indications. *J Clin Neurophysiol.* 2015;32: 87−95.
29. Alvarez V, Lee JW, Westover MB, et al. Therapeutic coma for status epilepticus: differing practices in a prospective multicenter study. *Neurology.* 2016;87:1650−1659.
30. DeLorenzo RJ, Hauser WA, Towne AR, et al. A prospective, population-based epidemiologic study of status epilepticus in Richmond, Virginia. *Neurology.* 1996,46. 1029−1035.
31. Tiamkao S, Pranboon S, Thepsuthammarat K, et al. Incidences and outcomes of status epilepticus in a 9-year longitudinal national study. *Epilepsy Behav.* 2015;49:135−137.
32. Legriel S, Bresson E, Deye N, et al. Cardiac arrest in patients managed for convulsive status epilepticus: characteristics, predictors, and outcome. *Crit Care Med.* 2018;46. [Epub ahead of print].
33. Hocker S, Prasad A, Rabinstein AA. Cardiac injury in refractory status epilepticus. *Epilepsia.* 2013;54:518−522.

CHAPTER 13

Simulating Encephalitis

Encephalitis presents variably with confusion, memory loss, psychiatric symptoms, and impaired consciousness, frequently punctuated by seizures and other manifestations depending on the cause. Acute encephalitis may progress over days, gradually adding to the constellation of symptoms and signs. Causes may be infectious, postinfectious, autoimmune, or paraneoplastic. Comprehensive supportive care maximizes the chance of a favorable outcome and involves management of neurologic sequelae. Some of these include severe uncontrollable agitation; movement disorders such as dystonia, dyskinesias, myoclonus, or seizures; and, in many of the autoimmune encephalitides, additional dysautonomia. Any of these manifestations—particularly when compromising airway, hemodynamics, patient or staff safety—may require admission to an intensive care unit.

There is some urgency with specific treatment of encephalitis. Encephalitis is often empirically treated with antiviral drugs. In patients where there is a high suspicion of autoimmune encephalitis, early immunotherapy confers a better treatment outcome than delayed therapy,[1–3] and early recognition and treatment of cancer improves outcomes in paraneoplastic encephalitis. Simulating a presentation of acute encephalitis—with quite specific approaches in some types—is therefore an important part of an acute neurology curriculum.

This scenario involves the clinical recognition of acute encephalitis and the actions (i.e., neuroimaging, laboratory evaluation, empiric treatment, and supportive care) required to achieve the best possible outcome. While nothing replaces the experience of seeing patients firsthand, simulating a tachycardic patient who has been intubated for control of severe agitation approaches the experience to a far greater degree than other methods of teaching.

THE PROBLEM BEFORE US

Acute encephalitis presents with confusion followed by a decline in the level of consciousness and is often accompanied by focal or generalized seizures and fever. The differential diagnosis is broad and must be narrowed focusing on treatable causes, as time to initiation of targeted treatment may mean the difference between recovery and persistent disability or death. The physician must first focus on stabilization, obtaining historical data and physical clues to narrow the etiologic possibilities, and initiating empiric treatment for Herpes simplex virus, before proceeding to the diagnostic evaluation.

Essential questions helpful in narrowing the differential diagnosis include recent vaccination or travel, animal contact (especially bats or other wild animals), tick or mosquito exposure, immunosuppression, IV drug use, or other channels of exposure to HIV. Geographical location and time of year can also help to narrow the possibilities; certain infectious causes of encephalitis are typically localized to specific geographic regions and seasons as a result of their method of transmission.[3–5] Paraneoplastic or autoimmune-mediated limbic encephalitis should be considered when infectious causes seem highly unlikely and the patient has other suggestive features. Unfortunately, the cancer is identifiable in only a small subset of patients; thus, PET scans are obligatory when risk factors are present (e.g., smoking, family history).

Patients should receive empiric treatment with IV acyclovir to treat encephalitis caused by HSV 1 and HSV 2 before diagnostic evaluation and within hours of presentation. Diagnostic evaluation should include neuroimaging regardless of whether the patient has focal findings on examination because a structural lesion can present as an acute confusional state. Laboratory studies may be tailored to the individual patient after consideration of demographics and risk factors, but most viral serum and CSF panels cast a wide net (and an unexpected viral infection may be found).

Neurologic sequelae of encephalitis may include agitation, psychosis, coma, cerebral edema, seizures, movement disorders, dysautonomia-related hyperthermia, hemodynamic changes, profuse secretions, or hypoventilation. These are all easily recognizable with the exception of seizures, which may require EEG monitoring for diagnosis. Encephalitis is known for its association with systemic complications, including hyponatremia, hypoxemia, and hypotension, and all require rapid correction to avoid additional brain injury or confounding neurologic examinations. Fever and hyperthermia may result from infection, dysautonomia, or hypothalamic involvement. Whatever the mechanism of hyperthermia, it must be treated aggressively as it is both epileptogenic and may worsen cerebral edema through increasing the metabolic demand of the brain. Comprehensive supportive care can improve outcomes in acute encephalitis, and patients may rehabilitate nicely if they survive and are given the chance.[6-11]

Diagnostic criteria for encephalitis of a presumably infectious or autoimmune cause have been proposed, but it is far from certain if their application will increase detection by the general physician. A required major criterion is altered mental status (defined as decreased or altered level of consciousness or personality change) lasting 24 h or more with no alternative cause identified. Minor criteria, two of which are required for a possible diagnosis and three or more for a confirmed diagnosis, include documented fever, $\geq 38°C$ (100°F) within 72 h of presentation (before or after); generalized or partial seizures not fully attributable to a preexisting seizure disorder; new onset of focal neurologic findings; cerebrospinal fluid WBC count $\geq 5/mm^3$; and an EEG abnormality consistent with encephalitis, not attributable to another cause.[12]

The diagnosis of autoimmune encephalitis has increased over time.[13] Anti-NMDA receptor encephalitis predominantly affects children and young adults, and 80% of patients are female. It is one of the more clinically recognizable, immune-mediated encephalitis syndromes, presenting with progressively abnormal behavior, cognitive dysfunction, speech changes, seizures, movement disorders, reduced level of consciousness, autonomic dysfunction, and central hypoventilation.[2] It can occur with or without an associated neoplasm (typically ovarian teratoma). Treatment, including tumor resection, immunotherapy with corticosteroids, IV immunoglobulin, or plasma exchange, leads to substantial recovery in over 75% of patients, but many patients will be treated with rituximab.[1] Treatment with intravenous rituximab can be initiated as soon as infection (e.g., hepatitis C and tuberculosis) has been excluded.

THE PRESENTING CLINICAL PROBLEM

The parents of a 32-year-old woman with no psychiatric history called 911 because she displayed progressive anxiety, disorientation, and acting-out behavior. She was intubated in the field after her violent movements and agitation were refractory to lorazepam and haloperidol. The progressive and severe nature of her symptoms in the absence of any prior psychiatric history should

prompt consideration of acute encephalitis. The learner should tailor the history toward identifying treatable causes and consider new psychiatric disease as a diagnosis of exclusion. The learner should then complete a rapid diagnostic evaluation and initiate empiric antiviral therapy. The main objectives of this scenario are to (1) recognize encephalitis, (2) proceed quickly through a number of important diagnostic and therapeutic steps, and (3) manage the numerous sequelae of acute encephalitis. Key competencies of this scenario are summarized in Fig. 13.1, and learning objectives are listed in Table 13.1.

Preparation

It is difficult to realistically simulate severe agitation necessitating pharmacologic intervention without producing actor fatigue so we present a patient (mannequin) who has already been intubated and sedated for behavioral control. The mannequin is placed in a hospital bed in the ED with a peripheral IV inserted and vital signs showing on the monitor. It is connected to a mechanical ventilator on a controlled mode of ventilation. Before the simulation, learners will receive guidelines on the management of encephalitis.[14,15] Additional setup and equipment required are detailed in Table 13.2.

COACHING ACTORS

The role of parent is to provide information requested by the learner using a script that lists all relevant history and to answer negatively any question in which the answer is not provided in the script. The ED nurse acts as the confederate, describing the examination in response to the learner's maneuvers, administering medications as requested by the learner, and providing results when instructed by the facilitator (Table 13.3).

THE IDEAL LEARNER

L enters and makes introductions to *CONF* and *P*'s parent after seeing the ED Face Sheet. *CONF* reports that *P* has been sedated with propofol because when it is withheld even briefly, she becomes combative. *P*'s parent describes a 5-day history of progressive anxiety followed by disorientation over the last 48 h punctuated at times by spells of laughter and crying and, at other times, by head turning and twisting of the mouth. On direct questioning, the mother denies any history of seizures, substance abuse, recent infections, travel, vaccinations, exposures, recent major stressors, and prescription, illicit drug, or alcohol use. *L* then considers the possibility of intoxication,

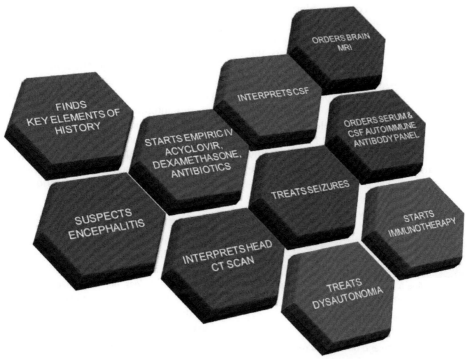

FIG. 13.1 Deconstruction of key competencies in encephalitis.

TABLE 13.1 Objectives
• Demonstrate focused history-taking skills in the setting of acute encephalitis
• Diagnose acute encephalitis
• Rapidly direct an appropriate initial diagnostic evaluation
• Initiate empiric treatment with intravenous acyclovir and immunotherapy when appropriate
• Recognize and manage the neurologic and systemic sequelae of acute encephalitis

TABLE 13.2 Simulation Scenario Setup for Encephalitis	
People needed	• Actor to play ED nurse • Actor to play parent • Attending or neurocritical care fellow to facilitate • Simulation technician to control the monitor

Equipment needed	• Ancillary tests
	  • Actual imaging results of a real patient brain CT and MRI
	  • Laboratory results on a separate sheet
	  • ECG
	• Syringes
	• Intravenous access
	• Blood pressure cuff
	• Mechanical ventilator, endotracheal tube

Setup needed	• ED Face Sheet in folder attached to door • Monitor showing tachycardia, arterial line reading mildly increased blood pressure • SimMan 3G on hospital bed, intubated and mechanically ventilated

encephalitis, or a structural lesion as the cause of severe agitation. *L* notes the fever and sinus tachycardia on the monitor. She asks *CONF* to give an additional liter of normal saline and to treat the fever with 1 g of acetaminophen and a cooling blanket. *L* then examines the patient and finds mydriasis, midline gaze, and intact brainstem reflexes. However, during examination (as a sign of dysautonomia), there is a several-second, self-limited run of supraventricular tachycardia with a heart rate in the 170's.

L requests blood cultures, complete blood count, chemistry, coagulation panel, drug of abuse screen, alcohol level, and a noncontrast head CT scan. Before the patient goes to the CT scanner, *L* requests the administration of IV acyclovir, ceftriaxone, vancomycin, and dexamethasone. *L* reviews the CT scan (normal) and laboratory results (normal). After *P* returns from the CT scan, *L* performs a spinal fluid examination and inquires about the color of the fluid (clear) and the opening pressure (11 cm H$_2$O). *L* strongly suspects an autoimmune cause, specifically anti-NMDA receptor encephalitis, and states that he must first confirm that CSF is consistent with the diagnosis and, specifically, that the gram stain and HSV PCRs are negative. *CONF* provides *L* with the CSF

analysis (nucleated cells 135 [94% lymphocytes], erythrocytes 3, protein 50, glucose 58, gram stain negative). *L* then requests an EEG to rule out nonconvulsive seizures and a brain MRI. EEG (Fig. 13.2), and MRI (Fig. 13.3) are provided. On reviewing these studies, he orders administration of 4 mg IV lorazepam, 30 mg/kg of IV valproate, high-dose IV methylprednisolone, and autoimmune antibody panels in both serum and CSF. *L* diagnoses encephalitis, admits the patient to the neurointensive care unit, and gives admission orders including 1000 mg IV methylprednisolone, propranolol for treatment of possible dysautonomia and continuous EEG monitoring. Scenario ends.

THE NOT-SO-IDEAL LEARNER

Simulation of encephalitis may cause learners to make a number of diagnostic and management errors, mostly as a result of being unfamiliar with this unusual disorder.

1. *The learner does not recognize new-onset psychiatric disease as a first sign of encephalitis.* With an increase in the frequency of autoimmune encephalitis, the learner should know that presenting symptoms often fall within the psychiatric realm. This has to be appreciated early because it requires sending off CSF samples for specific auto antibodies, which can be very low and thus undetectable in serum.

TABLE 13.3
Instructions to Actors Before Simulation

- Simulated patient is a mannequin, which allows portrayal of marked changes in vital signs.
- Spouse provides history details of anxiety, disorientation, and psychotic behavior.
- Nurse is present to guide and obtain test results.
- Nurse may ask prodding questions about the diagnosis.

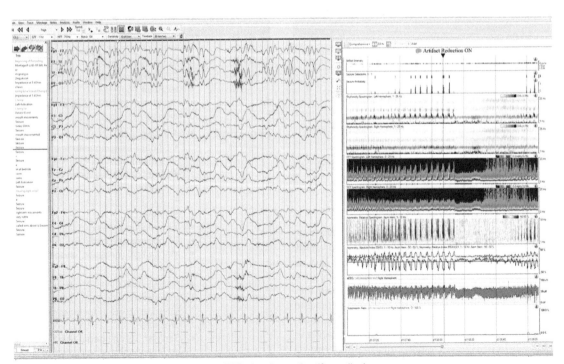

FIG. 13.2 EEG showing epileptiform discharges.

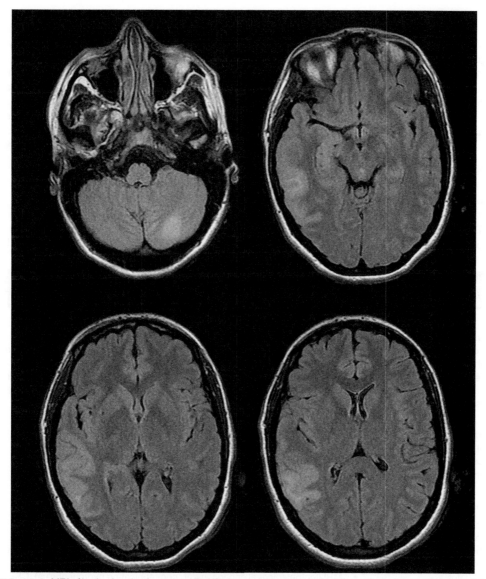

FIG. 13.3 MRI of brain showing increased FLAIR signal abnormality in the left cerebellar hemisphere and right temporal and parietal lobes with associated enlargement of the gyri in a patient with NMDA receptor encephalitis.

2. *The learner delays or does not administer IV acyclovir.* There is some urgency because delay may worsen outcome. The data are not clear on how long a delay is acceptable before the virus creates permanent havoc. Many emergency physicians start IV acyclovir while awaiting the PCR, and there is no harm doing that.

3. *The learner does not consider nonconvulsive seizures.* This is a frequent oversight; patients may be seizing before it becomes obvious clinically. Continuous EEG will be able to demonstrate epileptic discharges that require treatment if there is a clear clinical correlation.

4. *The learner ignores dysautonomia.* These manifestations can be substantial and involve changes in vital signs such as heart rate, blood pressure, and secretions. Many patients will have a baseline tachycardia and episodes of hypertension, and all can be treated with standard drugs such as beta blockade.

5. *The learner does not appreciate the need for aggressive immunosuppressive therapy.* Again, with the major epidemiologic shift of "unexplained viral encephalitis" to autoimmune encephalitis, early treatment with corticosteroids and intravenous immunoglobulin or plasma exchange should be considered in highly suspicious cases (e.g., female with psychosis of acute onset). Extensive evaluation for possible ovarian teratoma is needed to treat the source.

ADAPTING THE SCENARIO

This scenario is designed for learners with a background in neurology. It can be made less challenging by removing any one aspect (e.g., dysautonomia or seizures). The scenario is easily adapted for learners in the fields of emergency medicine, critical care, internal medicine or family practice, and psychiatry. The difficulty level can be altered to challenge a range of learners, from interns to practicing physicians. Any type of encephalitis can be written into a scenario. Possible adaptations include infectious, postinfectious, history and evaluation only, and more complex scenarios such as LGI1 presenting with limbic encephalitis intubated for severe agitation and complicated by severe hyponatremia,[16] herpes simplex encephalitis with a swollen temporal lobe,[17] or acute disseminated encephalomyelitis[18] complicated by severe cerebral edema.

DEBRIEFING

The debriefing can be used to discuss options for management of agitation in this setting, as well as to review the differential diagnosis and evaluation (Table 13.4).

TABLE 13.4
Differential Diagnosis of Acute Encephalitis[1]

Disorder	Diagnostic Studies
Demyelinating/Inflammatory • Acute disseminated encephalomyelitis • Neurosarcoidosis • Tumefactive multiple sclerosis/neuromyelitis optica	• Preceding infection or vaccination; MRI with diffuse, multifocal, poorly demarcated lesions predominantly involving white matter • Hilar adenopathy or pulmonary parenchymal changes, elevated ACE level (nonspecific) • CSF oligoclonal bands (nonspecific), lesions separated in time and space, NMO antibodies
Infectious • Bacterial encephalitis • Fungal infection • Spirochetal encephalitis • Viral encephalitis	• CSF testing: Cultures, AFB smear, Multiple PCR's HSV1/2, HHV6, VZV, EBV, CMV. HIV, VDRL, Lyme antibodies, arbovirus panel, enterovirus PCR • Serum testing: HIV, Lyme serology • Travel and exposure history
Inherited • Mitochondrial cytopathies	• Serum or CSF lactate elevation, lactate peak on MR spectroscopy
Neoplastic • Diffuse glioma • Lymphoma • Leptomeningeal carcinomatosis	• MRI (expansile, T2 hyperintense lesion), normal CSF • MRI (parenchymal or leptomeningeal enhancement); CSF cytology, flow cytometry, and IgH gene rearrangement • MRI (leptomeningeal enhancement, communicating hydrocephalus), CSF cytology
Toxicity and Deficiencies • Adverse reaction to psychotropics • Intoxication • Carbon monoxide poisoning • Wernicke encephalopathy	• Causative medications (e.g., neuroleptics, antiemetics), dopaminergic withdrawal, elevated creatine kinase • Serum and urine toxicology screens • Exposure • Alcohol misuse or malnutrition, oculomotor dysfunction, MRI (periaqueductal gray, mammillary bodies, medial thalami)
Vascular • Behçet disease • Posterior reversible encephalopathy syndrome • Primary or secondary angiitis of the CNS • Susac syndrome	• Painful mucocutaneous ulcers, uveitis • Headaches, hypertension, causative medications (e.g., immunosuppression, angiogenesis inhibitors), MRI (posterior predominant or brainstem T2 hyperintensities) • Abnormal vascular imaging, ANCA, cryoglobulins, aPL antibodies • Hearing loss, branch retinal artery occlusions on fluorescein angiography, MRI (corpus callosum and periventricular white matter abnormalities)

Specifically, the debriefing should emphasize early treatment with IV acyclovir and early initiation of immunotherapy in suspected postinfectious or antibody-mediated encephalitis after exclusion of infection. An important discussion point is the common concern of increased intracranial pressure (ICP) in patients with encephalitis, highlighting that increased ICP is most commonly seen in HSV or postinfectious encephalitis, where mass effect may prompt decompressive surgery. Additional time is devoted to discussion of neurologic and systemic sequelae and their management.

CONCLUSIONS

Through this simulation, learners can independently diagnose and direct the evaluation and management of acute encephalitis. Several medical complications pertinent to encephalitis can occur such as agitation, dysautonomia, and laboratory abnormalities, all of which require urgent treatment. Seizures are common in HSV and autoimmune encephalitis and, in fact, often determine the outcome. Successful treatment of encephalitis in young people requires a major team effort.

REFERENCES

1. Dalmau J, Lancaster E, Martinez-Hernandez E, et al. Clinical experience and laboratory investigations in patients with anti-NMDAR encephalitis. *Lancet Neurol.* 2011;10: 63−74.
2. Graus F, Titulaer MJ, Balu R, et al. A clinical approach to diagnosis of autoimmune encephalitis. *Lancet Neurol.* 2016;15:391−404.
3. McKeon A. Paraneoplastic and other autoimmune disorders of the central nervous system. *Neurohospitalist.* 2013;3:53−64.
4. El Khoury MY, Hull RC, Bryant PW, et al. Diagnosis of acute deer tick virus encephalitis. *Clin Infect Dis.* 2013;56: e40−e47.
5. Mostashari F, Bunning ML, Kitsutani PT, et al. Epidemic West Nile encephalitis, New York, 1999: results of a household-based seroepidemiological survey. *Lancet.* 2001;358:261−264.
6. Halperin J, ed. *Encephalitis: Diagnosis and Treatment.* New York: Informa Healthcare; 2007.
7. Nakano A, Yamasaki R, Miyazaki S, et al. Beneficial effect of steroid pulse therapy on acute viral encephalitis. *Eur Neurol.* 2003;50:225−229.
8. Ramos-Estebanez C, Lizarraga KJ, Merenda A. A systematic review on the role of adjunctive corticosteroids in herpes simplex virus encephalitis: is timing critical for safety and efficacy? *Antivir Ther.* 2014;19:133−139.
9. Singh TD, Fugate JE, Hocker S, et al. Predictors of outcome in HSV encephalitis. *J Neurol.* 2016;263:277−289.
10. Singh TD, Fugate JE, Rabinstein AA. The spectrum of acute encephalitis: causes, management, and predictors of outcome. *Neurology.* 2015;84:359−366.
11. Widener RW, Whitley RJ. Herpes simplex virus. *Handb Clin Neurol.* 2014;123:251−263.
12. Venkatesan A, Tunkel AR, Bloch KC, et al. Case definitions, diagnostic algorithms, and priorities in encephalitis: consensus statement of the international encephalitis consortium. *Clin Infect Dis.* 2013;57:1114−1128.
13. Dubey D, Pittock SJ, Kelly CR, et al. Autoimmune encephalitis: epidemiology and a comparison to infectious encephalitis. *Ann Neurol.* 2018;83:166−177.
14. Solomon T, Michael BD, Smith PE, et al. Management of suspected viral encephalitis in adults−Association of British Neurologists and British Infection Association National Guidelines. *J Infect.* 2012;64:347−373.
15. Tunkel AR, Glaser CA, Bloch KC, et al. The management of encephalitis: clinical practice guidelines by the Infectious Diseases Society of America. *Clin Infect Dis.* 2008;47: 303−327.
16. Wang M, Cao X, Liu Q, et al. Clinical features of limbic encephalitis with LGI1 antibody. *Neuropsychiatr Dis Treat.* 2017;13:1589−1596.
17. Adamo MA, Deshaies EM. Emergency decompressive craniectomy for fulminating infectious encephalitis. *J Neurosurg.* 2008;108:174−176.
18. Ahmed AI, Eynon CA, Kinton L, et al. Decompressive craniectomy for acute disseminated encephalomyelitis. *Neurocrit Care.* 2010;13:393−395.

CHAPTER 14

Simulating Acute Spinal Cord Compression

Compression of the spinal cord remains one of the most important neurologic emergencies because of the very real and significant potential for irreversible injury, particularly with the passage of time.[1–3] Acute spinal cord compression is usually seen under three circumstances—compression from cancer, blood, or abscess. First, it is fairly quickly appreciated in any patient with new leg weakness and prior metastasis of a known cancer. But in the other two situations, the presentation can be more difficult to recognize. Astute clinicians may suspect the development of an acute epidural hematoma in anticoagulated patients with significant thoracic or lumbar pain, but the most difficult-to-recognize type of spinal cord compression is the patient who presents mainly with sepsis and progressive hypotension. In those patients, septic shock is in the forefront, including resuscitative fluid and vasopressor management, and recognizing the additional presence of spinal cord injury depends on the physician's level of experience, vigilance, and dissatisfaction with an unresolved clinical problem. Of course, spinal cord compression is serious, and the spinal cord cannot sustain many hours of acute compression. Therefore, these disorders matter,[4] and it is important to offer a simulation scenario involving spinal cord compression.

In this chapter, we describe a simulation scenario in which a patient with an epidural abscess presents with sepsis. Sepsis compromises its clinical recognition.

THE PROBLEM BEFORE US

Spinal epidural abscess may present distinctly from other causes of spinal cord compression. Some patients are clearly at risk such as those with a recent spinal surgical procedure, indwelling spinal hardware, diabetes mellitus, intravenous drug use, chronic liver or kidney disease, and other known sites of infection. Not uncommonly, vertebral osteomyelitis is seen in these patients, and some series have found evidence in nearly 80% of patients with epidural abscesses.[5,6] Epidural abscesses are more frequent in immunocompromised patients.

An epidural abscess usually occurs when bacteria are disseminated hematogenously to the epidural space. The posteriorly located thoracolumbar area, where the space is larger and which contains more fat, is far more likely to be the site of an abscess.

Back pain has been identified in approximately 90% of patients, but many may not volunteer that, due to frequent comorbid loss of mental clarity resulting from their systemic infection. Symptoms usually occur fairly rapidly, within a matter of days to a week, with back pain, fever, and then a phase often characterized by radiculopathy with radiating pain and tingling. Fever is present in approximately two-thirds of the patients but less often in immunocompromised patients and patients with prior IV drug use.[5]

Clinical features of epidural spinal abscess correspond to its localization. Most often, limbs are initially flaccid and areflexic. There may also be relative hypotension that can be attributed to spinal shock or to early sepsis symptomatology. In many instances, conus and cauda equina symptomatology is seen, typically showing paraparesis, loss of sphincter function, and loss of sensation in several lumbar dermatomes with a sensory level at the waist. Cauda equina also shows reduced sensation from the sacral saddle region and further in the groin area.

Patients with an epidural abscess can present with sepsis and sepsis syndrome that may cause physicians to focus on treating the sepsis without further investigation of the source in the spinal canal. Alternatively, hypotension may be misinterpreted as part of dysautonomia with acute spinal shock, and resulting in inadequate fluid resuscitation. An astute physician observes weakness in both legs, abnormal sensation in the buttock area, and abnormal sphincter function to arrive at the diagnosis of spinal abscess.

A regular X-ray of the thoracolumbar spine might indicate initial evidence of a vertebral osteomyelitis, but in most instances, it is normal. An MRI scan, preferably with gadolinium administration, will show multiple different patterns, where multiple enhancing collections can be found with a decreased signal on T1 images and increased signal on T2 images. Several of these collections can be spread out through the epidural canal, or a large local collection compresses the cord. In many instances, *Staphylococcus aureus*, both methicillin-resistant (MRSA) and methicillin-sensitive (MSSA) organisms, can be identified as the pathogen-causing epidural abscesses. Many patients have abnormal erythrocyte sedimentation and C-reactive protein up to a point that normal results would make the presence of a spinal epidural abscess far less likely.

After the diagnosis is made, a neurosurgeon will determine whether decompression through laminectomy can be achieved or antibiotic treatment is a better option. Extensive abscesses spread out through longer trajectories are not surgically feasible, and antibiotics alone could be the only option for these patients. Surgery is often considered if there is significant pain or progressive neurologic deficit despite antibiotics, but in many patients with complete loss of function, decompressive surgery, which consists of irrigation and culture of the pathogen, will be performed.[5–9] In other words, the need for early recognition and management is self-evident with outcome clearly linked to time

to treatment. Management of these patients involves early intravenous antibiotics and securing vital signs. In a patient presenting with sepsis and risk of further ischemic compromise in an already compressed spinal cord, it is advisable to ensure adequate mean arterial blood pressures to support spinal cord perfusion.

THE PRESENTING CLINICAL PROBLEM

The setting here is a patient, played by an actor, presenting with septic shock and then, upon more detailed evaluation, a paraparesis. Vital signs on the monitor suggest an inflammatory state, and laboratory results indicate an increased white blood cell count and a mild lactic acidosis.

The patient is a 40-year-old man with a history of alcohol and drug abuse, who has had malaise and extreme fatigue, barely managing to get out of bed for the last 5 days. His wife often noticed him sweating at night but is not sure if he was febrile. He has recently begun to cough. The key competencies are shown in Fig. 14.1. The objectives are listed in Table 14.1. The main challenge is to link an ongoing infection with a spinal cord abscess.

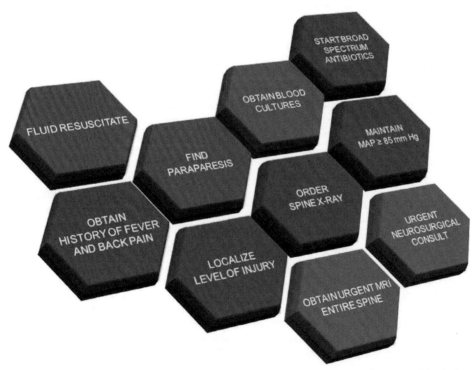

FIG. 14.1 Deconstructing key competencies in acute spinal cord compression from an epidural abscess presenting with early sepsis.

TABLE 14.1 Objectives
• Diagnose sepsis and initiate sepsis protocol (Table 14.5) • Localize paraparesis and sensory level • Initiate a search for the cause of epidural abscess • Order appropriate neuroimaging and interpret MRI correctly • Request neurosurgery evaluation • Consider corticosteroids

TABLE 14.2 Scenario Setup for Spinal Cord Compression	
People needed	• Actor to play the patient • Actor to play the nurse • Attending or neurocritical care fellow to facilitate
Equipment needed	• Syringes • Blood pressure cuff • Intravenous access • Reflex hammer • Laboratory results
Setup needed	• Monitor showing sinus rhythm, BP 90/50 mmHg, heart rate 100 bpm, mildly increased respiratory rate, normal SpO$_2$ on room air, temperature 39°C • Patient in hospital bed with peripheral IV catheter inserted and BP cuff/telemetry leads attached • Imaging to interpret (monitor off): • X-ray spine, X-ray chest, MR spine

BP, blood pressure; *IV*, intravenous; *SpO$_2$*, peripheral capillary oxygen saturation.

Preparation

The patient is lying in bed in the emergency department. The monitor shows a blood pressure of 90/50 mmHg, heart rate of 100 beats/min, and respiratory rate of 30. Temperature is 39°C. A few needle marks are applied with moulage in the antecubital fossa. The learner has the opportunity to request imaging studies, including a regular spine image as well as a chest X-ray, and later, when the diagnosis of spinal cord compression is considered, an MRI scan. All images are available in the room. The scenario setup is shown in Table 14.2.

Coaching Actors

Instructions to the actor are shown in Table 14.3. An actor can easily simulate paraparesis. This also applies to sensory loss from the waist to the navel. Actors may be able to suppress reflexes by not relaxing muscles. If asked, the actor should tell the learner that he is unable to void. It is possible to portray neck stiffness by wincing and stiffening when the neck is moved in the anterior-to-posterior direction and relaxing when it is moved laterally and confusion by answering erratically and appearing disoriented in time and place.

THE IDEAL LEARNER

L enters the emergency department and receives a face sheet that provides basic vitals and laboratory values. *L* enters and *CONF* will say: "this patient was transferred with fever and considerable confusion, and the provider thought he may have some weakness. He has had a soft blood pressure since he has been here."

L first identifies that *P* is possibly septic and initiates severe sepsis and septic shock activation. This includes ordering several labs, including lactate and blood cultures, and initiating antibiotics (Table 14.4). *L* also administers a bolus of 500 cc normal saline, assesses the response, and considers a bedside ultrasound to evaluate inferior vena cava size and compressibility. An echocardiogram for right ventricle (RV) and left ventricle (LV) size and function should also be considered. When addressed, *P* will be confused and disoriented but not agitated. He is unable to provide a history. *P*'s spouse provides a history of general malaise, chills at night, and worsening of his long-standing low back pain. *CONF* will ask, "Why do you think he is septic?" This prompts *L* to obtain a chest X-ray, which shows no abnormalities. *L* then examines *P* and finds him confused and difficult to assess. He finds some neck stiffness but normal eye movements, no facial asymmetry, and no arm drift. *L* quickly identifies that *P* is barely moving his legs (only some contraction of the quadriceps but no major movements in joints) and proceeds with sensory testing. He concludes by finding a sensory level at the navel and a flaccid paraparesis. At that time, *P* complains that he needs to void, and *CONF* tells *L* that *P* has a demonstrably full bladder but could not void when attempting to use a portable urinal. *CONF* appears concerned and asks *P* why is he not moving his legs, at which point *L* concludes that *P* could have a spinal epidural abscess causing compression of the cord and orders an X-ray of the spine. This is displayed on the monitor and shows no abnormalities. *L* then orders an MRI scan. *CONF* tells him he

TABLE 14.3
Instructions to Actors Before Simulation
• Confused speech, e.g., "where am I?" "what is happening?" "I don't know," "I have pain everywhere."
• Move legs only minimally; ideally, try not to move them at all
• Display clear difference of sensation with pinprick at the navel level
• Display some neck stiffness
• If asked, say you cannot void

has to speak with the neuroradiologist on call. In a conversation with the neuroradiologist (played by the instructor on the other line), he is given pushback, but *L* persists and explains that MRI is urgently indicated and should have priority over other cases. MRI shows a large, localized epidural abscess (Fig. 14.2). *L* contacts a neurosurgeon urgently, who will proceed with surgical evacuation. He maintains a MAP above 85 mmHg to avoid additional ischemic spinal cord injury from compression. Scenario ends.

THE NOT-SO IDEAL LEARNER

We anticipate the following errors in judgment will be made:

1. *The learner fixates on neck stiffness and thus considers acute bacterial meningitis.* He or she recognizes sepsis but considers the abnormality to be the result of meningitis and proceeds with a lumbar puncture, which will worsen the clinical features with full paraplegia.
2. *The learner treats sepsis inadequately.* The learner fails to fluid-resuscitate first and provides norepinephrine to maintain MAP >65 mmHg.
3. *The learner fails to consider source control.* The learner fails to recognize that low back pain might indicate vertebral osteomyelitis. Needle marks are not recognized despite clinical history of drug abuse. The patient is admitted to ICU delaying surgical treatment of the abscess.
4. *The learner fails to appreciate this is a neurosurgical emergency.* The learner may identify the abscess and start antibiotics but takes no further action.
5. *The learner fails to understand the urgency of neurosurgical decompression.* The learner does not attempt to convince the neuroradiologist that the patient has the utmost priority and may need urgent surgery, thus delaying MRI and spinal decompression.

ADAPTING THE SCENARIO

The scenario here involves epidural abscess presenting initially as sepsis. Depending on the learner, whether this is a practicing physician or trainee in general critical care, neurocritical care, or emergency medicine, more or less emphasis can be placed on recognition and management of the sepsis. The instructor can manipulate the vital signs to make the shock more or less severe and have the learner proceed with management including the type of fluid for resuscitation, type of vasopressors, and when to initiate mineralocorticoids or corticosteroids for refractory distributive shock.

DEBRIEFING

The debriefing includes first the diagnosis of paraparesis, location of the sensory level, and understanding and discussion of the neurologic features of spinal cord compression. Examination of spinal cord injury is largely classified on the basis of the severity of muscle involvement and weakness and the degree of sensory dysfunction. The American Spinal Cord Injury Association (ASIA) has classified the impairment from grade A to E (Table 14.6). Emphasis is on the clues including the combination of fever and focal neurologic deficits. The discussion can further extend toward explanation of how certain levels of compression affect the neurologic examination and how to explain specific neurologic deficits. A detailed discussion of spinal cord injury classification can follow. The discussion can also extend to risk factors for and causes of an epidural abscess and the importance of neuroimaging the entire spine. Debriefing should emphasize that in these situations, learners should understand that pushing for an MRI is essential in this diagnosis and to discuss how best to convince neuroradiologists to obtain an MRI scan urgently.

Debriefing can also discuss the neurosurgical options for these patients and the challenges in management. Antibiotic options are reviewed (Table 14.5), and indications for (or against) neurosurgical intervention are discussed.[10–12] Discussion of outcomes and the relationship between timely treatment and ultimate neurologic deficit should be emphasized. Debriefing may also discuss managing sepsis and initial course of action. The debriefing can start with a review of the management of sepsis. Topics to be covered include the following: How much fluid? When should a vasopressor be started and what should trigger the addition of a second? Which vasopressor should be used first and second? When are steroids beneficial? Finally, the use of steroids for spinal cord edema in the setting of epidural abscess is discussed to round out the body of knowledge needed to treat this disorder.

TABLE 14.4
Septic Shock Activation Protocol

Does your patient have two of the following? (Defines SIRS)	Action
Temperature >38°C or <36°C HR > 90 RR > 20 or PACO$_2$ < 34 WBC > 12,000 or <4000 or >10% immature bands	• Consider further evaluation for sepsis • Does this patient have risk factors, signs, or symptoms of infection?

Does your patient have SIRS and any of the following? (Defines SEPSIS)	
Hypotension Fever or hypothermia Tachycardia Tachypnea Leukocytosis leukopenia	• Lactate • Blood culture × 2 • Antibiotics (Table 11.4)

Does your patient have SEPSIS and organ dysfunction? (Defines SEVERE SEPSIS)

Lactate >4	Hypotension	

Other abnormalities

• Anion gap (>13)	• Hyperglycemia (>140)	• 30 mg/kg bolus
• Base excess (>4)	• Hypoxemia (PAO$_2$ < 60);	• Assess fluid response

• Increased INR (>1.5)	• Decreased urine output (<0.5 mL/kg/hr × 2 h)	• Bedside ultrasound:
		  • Vena cava size and variability
		  • Ventricular size and function

• Increased bilirubin (>2)	• Decreased platelets (<100K or 20K decrease from baseline)	
• Increased creatinine (>1.2)		

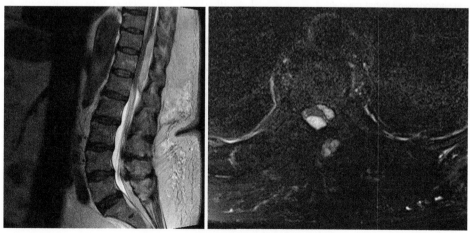

FIG. 14.2 Epidural abscess (T10 to L2).

TABLE 14.5
Antibiotics for Sepsis or Epidural Abscess

ANTIBIOTICS FOR SEPSIS

Vancomycin 25 mg/kg IV loading dose

Piperacillin/tazobactam 4.5 g IV q 8 h

Aztreonam 2 g IV q 8 h (if bactam allergy)

ANTIBIOTICS FOR EPIDURAL ABSCESS

Vancomycin 20 mg/kg IV q 8 h

Cefotaxime 2 g IV q 6 h or Nafcillin
(for Methicillin-sensitive Staphylococcus aureus [MSSA])

TABLE 14.6
ASIA Impairment Grading for Spinal Cord Injury

A	Complete	No motor or sensory function preserved in sacral (S4–S5) segments
B	Incomplete	Sensory but not motor function preserved below level including sacral (S4–S5) levels
C	Incomplete	Motor function preserved below level (more than half of key muscles and more than Medical Research Council [MRC] of 3)
E	Incomplete	Motor and sensory function normal

Proceed as follows:

- Determine sensory level (most caudal)
- Determine motor level (lowest key muscle of MRC ≥ 3)
- Determine complete or incomplete
- Designate as central cord, Brown-Séquard, anterior cord, conus medullaris, cauda equina

ASIA, American Spinal Injury Association.

CONCLUSIONS

Every year, patients with acute spinal cord compression are not recognized or are diagnosed too late leading to malpractice suits. Therefore, training to identify an acute spinal cord compression, including the cardinal findings of loss of spinal cord function, is important. Epidural abscess may present with sepsis or bacteremia and may catch physicians off guard. Simulation centers are ideal for recreating these circumstances.

REFERENCES

1. Cavaliere R, Schiff D. Epidural spinal cord compression. *Curr Treat Options Neurol.* 2004;6:285–295.
2. Ginsberg L. Disorders of the spinal cord and roots. *Pract Neurol.* 2011;11:259–267.
3. Ribas ES, Schiff D. Spinal cord compression. *Curr Treat Options Neurol.* 2012;14:391–401.
4. Ropper AE, Ropper AH. Acute spinal cord compression. *N Engl J Med.* 2017;376:1358–1369.
5. Johnson KG. Spinal epidural abscess. *Crit Care Nurs Clin North Am.* 2013;25:389–397.
6. Tang HJ, Lin HJ, Liu YC, et al. Spinal epidural abscess—experience with 46 patients and evaluation of prognostic factors. *J Infect.* 2002;45:76–81.
7. Baleriaux DL, Neugroschl C. Spinal and spinal cord infection. *Eur Radiol.* 2004;14(suppl 3):E72–E83.
8. Flanagan EP, Pittock SJ. Diagnosis and management of spinal cord emergencies. *Handb Clin Neurol.* 2017;140:319–335.
9. O'Phelan KH, Bunney EB, Weingart SD, et al. Emergency neurological life support: spinal cord compression (SCC). *Neurocrit Care.* 2012;17(suppl 1):S96–S101.
10. Thomson C. Spinal cord compression secondary to epidural abscess: the importance of prompt diagnosis and management. *BMJ Case Rep.* February 7, 2018.
11. Reihsaus E, Waldbaur H, Seeling W. Spinal epidural abscess: a meta-analysis of 915 patients. *Neurosurg Rev.* 2000;23:175–204.
12. Darouiche RO, Hamill RJ, Greenberg SB, et al. Bacterial spinal epidural abscess. Review of 43 cases and literature survey. *Medicine.* 1992;71:369–385.

CHAPTER 15

Simulating Acute Bacterial Meningitis

Acute bacterial meningitis often progresses to a fulminant form in which patients start to decline rapidly in their responsiveness and may even need intubation for airway protection. Acute bacterial meningitis is often first diagnosed in the emergency department, where all the action should be multidisciplinary with neurologists, infectious disease specialists, and otorhinolaryngologists. Acute bacterial meningitis is one of the neuroemergencies that is eminently treatable and leads to rapid improvement with early broad-spectrum antibiotics and dexamethasone. However, it has a poor outcome if intervention is delayed even by as little as several hours.

This potential neurocatastrophe is uncommon in adults. Recognition is even more difficult now that the incidence of adult community-acquired bacterial meningitis has decreased, mostly as a result of meningococcal vaccination. Without question, presentation remains difficult to grasp with often less than half of patients presenting with the clinical symptoms of fever, headache, neck stiffness, and impaired consciousness. Once the diagnosis appears highly probable, a stepwise approach is warranted. Simulating a patient presenting with acute bacterial meningitis, therefore, must be an integral part of the curriculum of acute neurology.

There is little evidence that management of acute bacterial meningitis in the emergency department has drastically improved over time, and physicians continue to struggle with the diagnosis.[1-3] This chapter emphasizes the right course of action, what diagnostic tests are needed, how to treat effectively, and which additional specialties should become involved. The scenario is designed for emergency physicians and neurologists in training, but is relevant also to internists and family practitioners as these patients may present initially to primary care or urgent care clinics.

THE PROBLEM BEFORE US

Acute bacterial meningitis tends to be community-acquired and due to *Streptococcus pneumoniae* or *Neisseria meningitidis*. Pneumococcal meningitis can be expected in patients over 65 years of age, but food-borne *Listeria monocytogenes* is also comparatively common in the elderly. Pneumococcal vaccines have reduced the risk of pneumococcal meningitis considerably. However, meningitis from *S. pneumoniae* remains a fatal disease in approximately one-third of the patients who contract it.

Bacterial meningitis usually presents with a decreased level of consciousness, and essentially, patients who are fully alert and communicative most likely are not in the throes of active bacterial meningitis. Headaches are variable and generally less severe than in, for example, subarachnoid hemorrhage. Fever is common but may be low grade or absent in patients who have been taking antibiotics for a prior infection. Typically, these are patients who have had pneumonia or mastoiditis treated with antibiotics. Seizures are uncommon at the onset of bacterial meningitis but may come later. In fact, patients who do present with seizures may have a different diagnosis, and an epidural abscess should be considered. Focal findings, such as aphasia, hemiparesis, facial asymmetry, or abnormal extraocular eye movements, are not expected in patients with acute bacterial meningitis, certainly not when seen within the first hours of presentation. Generally, the typical triad of fever, neck stiffness, and impaired consciousness is found in less than 50% of the patients if seen early.

The general consensus is to obtain blood cultures immediately on arrival in the emergency department followed by an urgent CT scan and lumbar puncture. However, any patient suspected of having bacterial meningitis should immediately receive broad-spectrum IV antibiotics and IV dexamethasone before proceeding with the CT scan and CSF examination. The European Society of Clinical Microbiology and Infectious Diseases (ESCMID) has recommended a door-to-antibiotic time of less than 1 h,[4] although this is far too optimistic and does not reflect actual practice according to recent surveys in Europe.[1-3]

There continues to be a discussion of whether CT scan is required in a patient with acute bacterial meningitis and whether obtaining a CT scan delays lumbar puncture and, thus, diagnostic confirmation. However, the CT scan can reveal a subdural empyema with mass effect or early cerebral edema, which may make the sudden removal of a large volume of CSF extremely dangerous for the patient. Multiple cases of significant worsening soon after a lumbar puncture have been described as a result of this action. Later deterioration may be attributed to fulminant meningitis with the development of cerebral edema.

Once a CT scan shows no evidence of structural lesions or early brain edema, the physician should proceed with a spinal fluid examination. The recognition of brain edema on CT can be difficult, particularly in younger individuals, where sulci are barely present and may falsely suggest early brain edema. Generally, brain edema should be suspected if the sylvian fissures cannot be visualized and if the ventricles are compressed. Obliteration of the basal cisterns is a late phenomenon, and when seen, most of those patients will have abnormal brainstem reflexes and, often, already fixed and dilated pupils. Such a fulminant form can be associated either with development of cerebral edema, development of acute hydrocephalus, or development of increased intracranial pressure from diffuse thrombophlebitis of the cerebral venous system.

Lumbar puncture will mostly identify an increased leukocyte count, usually >2000 cells/mm³, protein level >1000 mg/dL, a glucose level <40 mg/dL, and a ratio of CSF glucose to blood glucose of <0.2. The Gram stain is often positive, and cultures are important because they will, in most instances, identify *Streptococcus pneumonia* or other bacteria. In many patients, the organism will grow out of a blood culture (early or late), and this can be seen in patients without clinical features of sepsis. Although frequently omitted, an opening pressure should be obtained and fluid removed until the closing pressure is normal.

Current recommendations include use of IV ampicillin to cover for listeria in high-risk patients, specifically patients with alcohol-use disorder and malnutrition as well as any patient over age 60 years. The clinical complexity of this CNS infection is further detailed elsewhere.[5–10]

Fluid resuscitation should be started emergently with 1000–2000 mL of crystalloids over 30 min in patients who have developed sepsis in the setting of bacterial meningitis. The usual target is a mean arterial blood pressure of 75 mmHg. Serum lactate should be measured quickly, and is an important indicator of tissue perfusion. A serum lactic acid level >4 mmol/L indicates tissue hypoperfusion and calls for aggressive hemodynamic support. A patient with a normal lactate can be in the early stages of a severe sepsis but adequately perfused. The patient's urinary output needs to be closely monitored for the development of oliguria (less than 20 mL/h).

Norepinephrine is the initial vasopressor of choice. It may be supplemented with low-dose vasopressin if the blood pressure target is not achieved. Phenylephrine is not a good choice in septic shock because it can reduce cardiac output, and these patients may already have myocardial dysfunction. If the left ventricular ejection fraction is reduced on echocardiogram and shock persists, administration of inotropes such as dobutamine should be started. After the patient has been successfully resuscitated, fluid administration becomes conservative (i.e., fluid balance even to negative) the focus shifts to prevention of complications from fluid overload (principally related to capillary leak leading to pulmonary edema).

Patients with septic shock not quickly responding to these measures may be treated with corticosteroids and fludrocortisone; this combination reduces mortality in any patient in septic shock.[11] Corticosteroids may reduce vasopressor dependency but do not appear to improve survival.

THE PRESENTING CLINICAL PROBLEM

A 60-year-old man with a prior history of alcohol abuse disorder presents to the emergency department with confusion, headache, and ear pain. Such a presentation should rapidly cue toward bacterial meningitis. The learner should recognize and manage the early presentation of acute bacterial meningitis, obtain a history of otitis media, and consider several possibilities for a decreased level of consciousness. The learner should recognize neck stiffness and do the appropriate test to find this important clinical sign.

The main objectives of this scenario are to (1) recognize bacterial meningitis, (2) proceed quickly with a number of important diagnostic and therapeutic steps, (3) obtain consultations from infectious disease and otorhinolaryngology, and (4) manage the sequelae of bacterial meningitis. The objectives are summarized in Table 15.1 and the key competencies in Fig. 15.1.

TABLE 15.1
Objectives

- Recognize the meningitis triad of fever, decreased consciousness, and neck stiffness
- Treat early signs of sepsis
- Use an appropriate sequence to treat and obtain test results
- Order antibiotics and dexamethasone before lumbar puncture
- Consider symptomatic hydrocephalus
- Consult otorhinolaryngology for mastoiditis

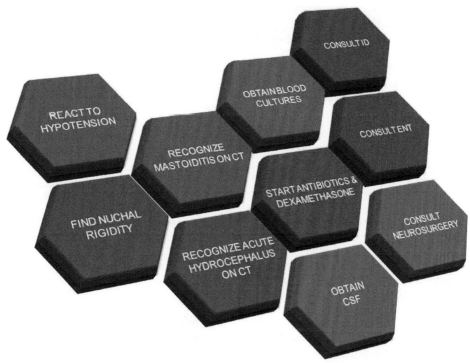

FIG. 15.1 Deconstructing key competencies in bacterial meningitis.

Preparation

The actor is placed in the hospital bed in the emergency department with peripheral IV inserted and vital signs showing early tachypnea, fever, and mild hypotension with a systolic blood pressure of 90 mmHg. Ideally, before the simulation, the learners will have received a paper on recognition and diagnosis of stupor and coma. In addition, the practice guidelines for management of bacterial meningitis are provided.[4] The scenario setup is shown in Table 15.2.

Coaching Actors

Suggestions for the actor are shown in Table 15.3. Simple instructions for the actor include sparse conversation with single syllables and displaying a fluctuating level of consciousness by falling asleep when not directly addressed. The scenario can be made more complex by having the actor mimic a seizure. The learner needs to identify neck stiffness, so the actor should keep his neck stiff when the learner attempts flexion and to a lesser degree, rotation. The classic examination parameters should include the Brudzinski and Kernig signs

TABLE 15.2 Scenario Setup for Acute Bacterial Meningitis	
People needed	• Simulation technician to control monitor • Actor to play patient • Actor to play ED nurse • Attending or neurocritical care fellow to facilitate
Equipment needed	• Syringes for blood culture • BP cuff • IV catheter • Oxygen by nasal catheter • Intubation tray • BIPAP • Antibiotics, dexamethasone, saline • Laboratory results • CT scan
Setup needed	• Monitor showing regular rhythm, mild hypotension (SBP 90 mmHg), increased RR (20/min), SPO$_2$ 90% • CT scan available • Chest X-ray available

TABLE 15.3 Actor Instructions
• Confused speech, e.g., "don't know," "headache," "don't feel right"—restlessness, turning
• Falls asleep unattended
• Fixates neck when learner flexes it but allows some rotation
• Cannot extend knee with hip flexion (Kernig's sign)
• Flexes both knees somewhat with neck flexion (Brudzinski's sign)

TABLE 15.4 Key CSF Findings	
CSF	2000 cells/μL
Glucose	36 g/L
Protein	1000 g/L
Gram stain	Positive for gram positive cocci in pairs and chains
Pressure	Markedly elevated—jets out of needle
Color	Cloudy

that can be easily simulated. Passive extension of the knees with the hips flexed at 90 degrees (Kernig sign) results in expression of pain. Neck flexion results in flexion of the knees and hips (Brudzinski sign). The role of the facilitator is to provide a flow to the scenario and consistently ask the learner for the next possible step and how to proceed. If the learner considers a CT scan, a CT scan will be provided. If she considers a spinal fluid examination, a needle will be provided and the procedure simulated without actual puncture.

THE IDEAL LEARNER

L enters and introduces herself to P and CONF after seeing the ED Face Sheet. P states that he is not feeling well but does not provide any further history, even with appropriate questioning. L should consider the differential diagnosis of abnormal consciousness, and she may consider a structural lesion or intoxication as the cause of stupor. L recognizes that the patient is febrile and mildly hypotensive, noting a systolic blood pressure of 90 mmHg on the monitor, and asks CONF to give additional fluids to improve the blood pressure, whereupon the blood pressure corrects to 100 mmHg systolic. L then examines the patient and, finding neck stiffness, orders an urgent CT scan. Before performing a lumbar puncture, L checks laboratory results, including INR and platelets, to make sure the patient can safely undergo the procedure. During this time, P continues to exhibit fluctuating levels of consciousness. Before the patient goes through the CT scanner, L provides appropriate antibiotics and dexamethasone (Table 15.4). A CT scan is available demonstrating early hydrocephalus and the effacement of one of the mastoids indicative of a mastoiditis (Fig. 15.2). After P returns from the CT scan, L performs a spinal fluid examination and is told that the CSF is cloudy (Table 15.4). L diagnoses bacterial meningitis and admits the patient to the neurointensive

care unit; she but also contacts otorhinolaryngology, infectious disease, and a neurosurgeon for further consultation. She includes in her admission orders parameters for aggressive treatment of fever and orders continuous EEG monitoring. Scenario ends.

THE NOT-SO-IDEAL LEARNER

The following missteps have been identified:

1. *The learner does not consider symptomatic hydrocephalus.* Some learners may perform only a diagnostic lumbar puncture and not consider the possibility that hydrocephalus is contributing to the reduction in level of consciousness.
2. *The learner pursues an inadequate sequence of action.* The learner does not obtain blood cultures before antibiotic administration, waits for CSF confirmation before administering antibiotics, or does not proceed with a CT scan before spinal fluid examination.
3. *The learner does not recognize early sepsis.* The learner fails to appreciate early sepsis in the setting of bacterial meningitis and does not correct blood pressure with fluids or consider activation of a sepsis protocol.
4. *The learner responds too slowly.* Slow action on the part of the physician markedly delays treatment of the patient.
5. *The learner does not recognize the need for other consultations.* This means that the learner has not recognized mastoiditis and the need for an urgent mastoidectomy by ENT, or hydrocephalus and the possible need for lumbar or extraventricular drainage.

ADAPTING THE SCENARIO

This scenario lends itself to teaching a lumbar puncture. As alluded to in Chapter 2, lumbar-puncture simulators

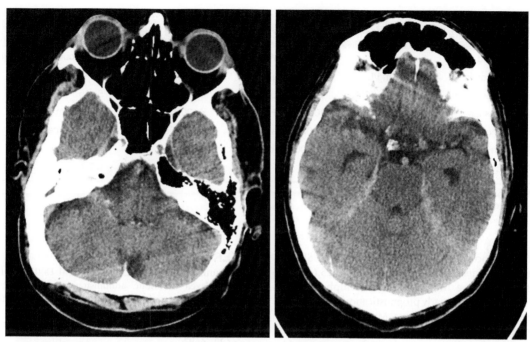

FIG. 15.2 CT scan: absence of air in the right mastoid indicative of mastoiditis on the right image and enlarged temporal horns on the left image indicating acute hydrocephalus.

TABLE 15.5
Advised Empiric Treatment for Adults With Community-Acquired Bacterial Meningitis[4]

Patient Group	Reduced *Streptococcus pneumoniae* Sensitivity to Penicillin	Normal *S. pneumoniae* Sensitivity to Penicillin
Age >18 and <50 years	Cefotaxime or ceftriaxone plus vancomycin or rifampicin	Cefotaxime or ceftriaxone
Age >50 years or age >18 and <50 years with risk factors for *Listeria monocytogenes*	Cefotaxime or ceftriaxone plus vancomycin or rifampicin plus amoxicillin/ampicillin/penicillin	Cefotaxime or ceftriaxone plus amoxicillin/ampicillin/penicillin

are commercially available and are quite valuable as teaching tools in all levels of training. The scenario can be further complicated by introducing seizures and worsening of respiratory parameters, which would require intubation. The scenario can be expanded using activation of a sepsis bundle (Chapter 14).

DEBRIEFING

The debriefing is used to discuss the recognition of bacterial meningitis, including the recent European guidelines in recognition and management, and which

steps to take for rapid management of bacterial meningitis.[4,9,12–15] A major emphasis is on early recognition and rapid administration of antibiotics (Table 15.5) and dexamethasone. A discussion of the evidence for IV dexamethasone on fulminant meningitis is important while also emphasizing the marked underutilization of IV dexamethasone in emergency room settings. Important teaching points should include evidence that untreated bacterial meningitis can lead to sepsis. Furthermore, the debriefing should cover the rationale for a CT scan (i.e., to exclude mass lesions such as abscess and subdural empyema and to

TABLE 15.6
Characteristics of Bacterial, Viral, and Tuberculous Meningitis[4]

Characteristic	Normal	Bacterial Meningitis	Viral Meningitis	Tuberculous Meningitis
C-reactive protein	<10 mg/L	40–400 mg/L	<10 mg/L	10–100 mg/L
Blood leukocytes	$4-10 \times 10^9/\mu l$	$10-30 \times 10^9/\mu L$	$4-10 \times 10^9/\mu L$	$5-15 \times 10^9/\mu L$
Opening pressure[b]	6–20 cm H_2O	20–50 cm H_2O	6–30 cm H_2O	15–40 cm H_2O
CSF[a] white cell count	<5 cells/μL	>1000 cells/μL	10–1000 cells/μL	10–1000 cells/μL
CSF protein level	60 mg/dL	>2000 mg/dL	60 mg/dL	1000 mg/dL
CSF/blood glucose ratio	>0.60	<0.40	>0.60	<0.40

[a] Cerebrospinal fluid.
[b] The pressure of CSF on lumbar puncture.

identify hydrocephalus). A brief discussion on CSF formula in CNS infections may follow (Table 15.6). It is worthwhile to use the debriefing to emphasize the need for caution with early prognostication, particularly if the patient presents with coma. Many patients recover remarkably well.

The debriefing also must emphasize how patients with meningitis can deteriorate (e.g., empyema, hydrocephalus, cerebral edema, seizures, hyperpyrexia, inadequate antimicrobial coverage) and how best to intervene. The rationale for otorhinolaryngology consultation (urgent mastoidectomy) and neurosurgical evaluation (worsening hydrocephalus) should be discussed. A discussion of the evidence for IV dexamethasone in pneumococcal meningitis is important while also stressing the marked underutilization of dexamethasone in emergency room settings.

CONCLUSION

Learners have the opportunity here not only to diagnose early bacterial meningitis but also to imprint in their memory the necessary steps to treat the condition quickly and appropriately. Early intracranial pressure monitoring, aggressive treatment of brain edema with high doses of corticosteroids, osmotic diuretics, decompressive craniectomy, and ventriculostomy for hydrocephalus are common interventions (and should be strongly considered), but there is no conclusive evidence of improved outcome. The most important variable is initial management and appropriate treatment with antibiotics within an hour of arrival in the emergency department.

REFERENCES

1. Auburtin M, Wolff M, Charpentier J, et al. Detrimental role of delayed antibiotic administration and penicillin-nonsusceptible strains in adult intensive care unit patients with pneumococcal meningitis: the PNEUMOREA prospective multicenter study. *Crit Care Med.* 2006;34: 2758–2765.
2. Bodilsen J, Brandt CT, Sharew A, et al. Early versus late diagnosis in community-acquired bacterial meningitis: a retrospective cohort study. *Clin Microbiol Infect.* 2018;24: 166–170.
3. Michael B, Menezes BF, Cunniffe J, et al. Effect of delayed lumbar punctures on the diagnosis of acute bacterial meningitis in adults. *Emerg Med J.* 2010;27:433–438.
4. van de Beek D, Cabellos C, Dzupova O, et al. ESCMID guideline: diagnosis and treatment of acute bacterial meningitis. *Clin Microbiol Infect.* 2016;22(suppl 3): S37–S62.
5. Brouwer MC, Wijdicks EF, van de Beek D. What's new in bacterial meningitis. *Intensive Care Med.* 2016;42: 415–417.
6. Muralidharan R, Mateen FJ, Rabinstein AA. Outcome of fulminant bacterial meningitis in adult patients. *Eur J Neurol.* 2014;21:447–453.
7. Muralidharan R, Rabinstein AA, Wijdicks EF. Cervicomedullary injury after pneumococcal meningitis with brain edema. *Arch Neurol.* 2011;68:513–516.
8. Rubin MN, Wijdicks EF. Fulminant streptococcal meningoencephalitis. *JAMA Neurol.* 2013;70:515.
9. van de Beek D, de Gans J, Tunkel AR, et al. Community-acquired bacterial meningitis in adults. *N Engl J Med.* 2006;354:44–53.
10. Vernino S, Wijdicks EF, McGough PF. Coma in fulminant pneumococcal meningitis: new MRI observations. *Neurology.* 1998;51:1200–1202.

11. Annane D, Renault A, Brun-Buisson C, et al. Hydrocortisone plus fludrocortisone for adults with septic shock. *N Engl J Med.* 2018;378:809−818.

12. Gerber J, Nau R. Mechanisms of injury in bacterial meningitis. *Curr Opin Neurol.* 2010;23:312−318.

13. McMillan DA, Lin CY, Aronin SI, et al. Community-acquired bacterial meningitis in adults: categorization of causes and timing of death. *Clin Infect Dis.* 2001;33.969−975.

14. van de Beek D, Brouwer M, Hasbun R, et al. Community-acquired bacterial meningitis. *Nat Rev Dis Primers.* 2016;2: 16074.

15. van de Beek D, Brouwer MC, Thwaites GE, et al. Advances in treatment of bacterial meningitis. *Lancet.* 2012;380: 1693−1702.

CHAPTER 16

Simulating Posterior Reversible Encephalopathy Syndrome

Posterior reversible encephalopathy syndrome (PRES) is an accepted term for a complex condition mostly associated with hypertensive crisis. The combination of hypertension and neurologic symptoms or signs is quite common in the emergency department but also in consultations of patients seen in surgical or medical intensive care units. Neurointensivists may also encounter the syndrome in their own patients in the context of hemodynamic augmentation for symptomatic vasospasm or in the setting of marked dysautonomia; for example, in patients with sympathetic overdrive in Guillain-Barre syndrome, acute spinal cord injury, or autoimmune encephalitis. In other words, PRES is seen with some regularity in hospital settings.

Abnormal content or level of consciousness, headache, seizures, and focal deficits are key features of PRES, but clinical symptomatology can vary widely. Recognition of PRES is important. It is often mistaken for delirium or encephalopathy due to a systemic infection, organ dysfunction, or drug, and thus the urgency goes unrecognized.

The resulting continued high blood pressures perpetuate the pathophysiology. In hypertensive crisis, there is virtually no controlled autoregulation in vascular beds, and therefore, an increase in blood pressure leads to endothelial injury as a result of mechanical stress. In addition, activation of the renin-angiotensin system leads to vasoconstriction and ischemia. This simulation scenario, therefore, can teach the clinical and CT scan findings of PRES and can test knowledge of the side effects of antihypertensives and potential consequences of over-aggressive treatment.

THE PROBLEM BEFORE US

Traditionally, hypertension has been defined as a systolic blood pressure >120 mmHg and a diastolic blood pressure >80 mmHg.[1] Hypertensive emergencies mostly require systolic blood pressures exceeding 180 mmHg or diastolic pressures exceeding 120 mmHg but are also defined by signs of end organ damage such as acute EKG changes, oliguria, or altered mental status. Hypertensive emergency is common in emergency departments, occurring in approximately one in four patients with known hypertension. Most patients have a history that includes long-standing hypertension and evidence of prior uncontrolled high blood pressure. There may also be recent concomitant use of nonsteroidal antiinflammatory drugs, which may increase intracranial pressure, or medication noncompliance due to poor access to care, health literacy, or loss of insurance. In many patients, there are other vascular risk factors such as hyperlipidemia, diabetes, obesity, and sleep apnea.

The pathophysiology of a hypertensive crisis is not fully understood; again most likely it is an autoregulation failure that increases vascular resistance followed by vasoconstriction, endothelial injury, ischemia, and end organ damage. There may also be an additional prothrombotic state or activation of a number of endothelial factors, causing increased vascular permeability and edema, particularly in end organs such as the brain and kidneys. Hypertensive emergency can also be seen in an acute aortic dissection or acute renal failure.

PRES refers to a disorder of vasogenic brain edema in patients with acute neurological symptoms, including headache, encephalopathy, seizures, and focal deficits, in the setting of a trigger such as acute severe hypertension, blood pressure fluctuations (e.g., in septic shock), cytotoxic drugs (typically cyclosporine or tacrolimus), autoimmune disorders, acute renal failure, and eclampsia.[2] The syndrome is usually reversible when the inciting factor is removed. PRES caused by acute severe hypertension is synonymous with what used to be called "hypertensive encephalopathy." The name PRES, however, is known to be a misnomer.[3] Many clinical and radiographic abnormalities are not predominantly in the posterior region, and some are not reversible and lead to true cerebral infarction or hemorrhage.[2,3] Furthermore, although encephalopathy is frequent, it is not universally present. Headache is nonspecific, but some patients may suffer a thunderclap headache at the onset of a hypertensive crisis. Visual disturbances may be as simple as blurred vision or visual field defects but can include cortical blindness with visual hallucinations. A minority of patients (10%−15%) have clear focal findings such as cortical blindness, hemiparesis, and aphasia. Seizures are common (occurring in up to 75% of patients) and can be focal or generalized.

The physical examination is important and should identify possible cardiac murmurs or abdominal murmurs for aortic dissection. Fundoscopy to assess for possible retinopathy may show flame hemorrhages, subconjunctival hemorrhages, and exudates or papilledema. The absence of pulses in the lower extremities, paraparesis, Horner's syndrome, and acute chest or back pain is highly suggestive of aortic dissection. Necessary ancillary tests include evaluation of cardiac biomarkers, renal indices, urinalysis (casts, proteinuria), electrocardiogram, and chest X-ray (to look for mediastinal widening, cardiac enlargement, or pulmonary edema). Hypertensive emergencies also present with some degree of pulmonary edema, and one in five patients may have evidence of myocardial injury or infarction.

The diagnosis is suspected clinically when there is definite cortical blindness or seizures in the setting of a hypertensive surge. PRES remains a clinical diagnosis, and patients may have normal neuroimaging despite having the classic risk factors and clinical syndrome. The severity of PRES on neuroimaging can be classified as mild (near-normal findings on MRI with some cortical or subcortical white-matter edema), moderate (confluent areas including the cerebellum, basal ganglia, and brainstem), and severe (involvement of multiple structures, often with associated petechial or subarachnoid hemorrhage,[4] mass effect, and evidence of cytotoxic edema on diffusion-weighted imaging[5,6]). Contrast enhancement may be gyriform or leptomeningeal and does not particularly portend a worse outcome.[7] In severe cases of PRES, cerebral vasoconstriction can be seen, often with multifocal patterns.[8,9] This vasoconstriction may explain the frequent involvement of the border zones between the anterior and middle cerebral artery and the middle and posterior cerebral artery territories. When restricted diffusion is present, it may indicate severe vasoconstriction that has led to infarction. Patients may have gadolinium enhancement, although gadolinium is rarely administered in patients with hypertensive crisis, who often also have an abnormal creatinine. Intracranial hemorrhage is seen in about one in four patients with PRES

and can appear in multiple compartments including the subarachnoid space.

The diagnosis of PRES can be made challenging by the fact that at-risk patients also typically have an illness related to multiorgan dysfunction, may be immunosuppressed, or have other risk factors for seizures and stroke. For this reason, patients with a clinical syndrome consistent with PRES frequently undergo lumbar puncture and CSF analysis to exclude CNS infection. CSF profiles in confirmed PRES have shown albuminocytologic dissociation with elevated protein levels and normal cells. Mild CSF pleocytosis can occur; however, it is uncommon and should prompt consideration of further testing for infectious or inflammatory causes.[10] Autoimmune encephalitis or lymphoma may have similar MRI profiles, particularly if abnormalities are progressive despite correction of hypertension. Hypoxemic-ischemic encephalopathy should be considered if there has been marked hypotension, respiratory or cardiac arrest, or septic emboli in the setting of endocarditis. It is important to consider other possibilities, which include encephalitis, CNS vasculitis, progressive multifocal leukoencephalopathy, osmotic demyelination syndrome in the setting of marked hyponatremia, or any toxic leukoencephalopathy (e.g., a history of illicit drug use). These alternative diagnoses are rare but should be considered in any patient with an unusual presentation or other clinical histories. PRES can also occur in the setting of an infection and sepsis. In that situation, the mechanism is likely different and associated with inflammatory endothelial damage and hypoperfusion.

Essentially, posterior reversible encephalopathy syndrome is a vascular leak syndrome in which hypertension pushes plasma through the blood-brain barrier and causes vasogenic brain edema. Further damage can cause ischemia resulting in cytotoxic edema, and both types can be differentiated on MRI.[2,11]

The general goal of blood pressure management in a crisis is to lower the blood pressure by approximately 10%−20% during the first hour of treatment. Blood pressure may be further lowered after that but by no more than 25% of the presenting pressure by the end of the first 24 h of treatment. Antihypertensive choices are based on rapidity of onset, half-life (drugs with shorter half-lives, such as clevidipine, nicardipine, fenoldopam, and nitroprusside, are more easily titratable), and patient comorbidities. For example, beta blockers may be avoided in heart block and vasodilators in aortic stenosis due to their significant afterload reduction. Typically, single doses of an IV drug, such as labetalol or hydralazine, are attempted and the response assessed. If multiple doses are required in a short period of time, continuous infusion of an IV anti-hypertensive agent, such as labetalol, esmolol, nicardipine, nitroprusside, or clevidipine, is initiated. Transitioning to an oral drug occurs after stabilization of the neurologic injury and control of hypertension. Oral regimens are often a combination of antihypertensives, and several can be considered. Generally first-line antihypertensive management is a thiazide diuretic, calcium-channel blocker, angiotensin-converting enzyme inhibitor, or angiotensin receptor blocker. Although normotension is the ultimate goal, it is rarely an appropriate goal while the patient remains in intensive care. The risks of overtreatment include induction of cerebral ischemia and infarction as the brain suddenly experiences a blood pressure well below its norm and/or acute tubular necrosis of the kidneys as they similarly experience a degree of perfusion well below previous levels.

THE PRESENTING CLINICAL PROBLEM

The actor plays a 75-year-old woman with a prior history of hypertension, on intermittent hemodialysis. Her blood pressure has always been difficult to control, and there are questions about her drug compliance. The patient has also been reluctant to undergo dialysis and skipped a recent session. She comes into the emergency department with marked loss of vision and a blood pressure of 250/160 mmHg. The actor displays no respiratory distress nor complaints of chest pain. The objectives here are to (1) recognize the neurologic findings including cortical blindness, (2) recognize seizure, (3) diagnose PRES, and (4) treat the hypertension and seizures (Table 16.1). Key competencies are shown in Fig. 16.1.

Preparation

An actor can easily portray the patient in this scenario, and the setting can be an emergency department. Two weeks before the simulation, learners receive a recent

---

TABLE 16.1
Objectives

- Recognize neurologic findings including cortical blindness
- Recognize seizure
- Diagnose PRES
- Safely treat the hypertension and seizures

---

review of PRES as part of the package. The scenario setup is shown in Table 16.2. Marked hypertension is shown on a monitor.

Coaching Actors

The actor is instructed not to blink to threat, not to fixate to testing of eye movements, and, when asked if she is able to see, to deny any problems with her vision. When asked what she sees, she confabulates, answering directed questions such as "what color is my tie?" erroneously but with confidence. The actor is coached to feign inability to track finger movements (Table 16.3). She should appear somewhat restless and inattentive (requiring repeated requests to perform a task) and then suddenly have a brief, generalized tonic-clonic seizure (initiated when the ER nurse taps her feet). The seizure resolves with brief snoring and a postictal state (portrayed as a lack of responsiveness with eyes closed).

The confederate in this scenario is the ED nurse. Specific instructions for this role include providing the medical history as relayed by paramedics and informing the learner when appropriate that the patient's medical record suggests a skipped dialysis session and includes documented medication noncompliance.

THE IDEAL LEARNER

L enters the simulation center and finds P in bed. L immediately identifies that P has a marked hypertension and, before he starts treating it, obtains a history from CONF, who explains the past medical history and multiple antihypertensives that have been prescribed with documented medication noncompliance. L asks for basic laboratory values, and they are provided. L then requests placement of an arterial line and proceeds to treat with antihypertensives. He starts with 10 mg IV labetalol and awaits the response. He explicitly states that the target will be to lower the systolic blood pressure to between 200 and 225 mmHg and when the goal is not reached with labetalol, starts, an infusion of IV nicardipine. L then examines P, noting a normal level of alertness, marked inattention, and cortical blindness. Considering a differential diagnosis of PRES, embolus to the basilar artery causing occipital infarcts, infectious or autoimmune encephalitis, and CNS vasculitis, he orders a head CT scan and asks CONF to set up for a lumbar puncture. CONF points L toward the head CT scan and taps the foot of the patient to induce a seizure. L quickly reviews the CT scan (Fig. 16.2) and identifies bilateral, asymmetric hypodensities consistent with vasogenic edema. He instructs CONF to give 2 mg IV

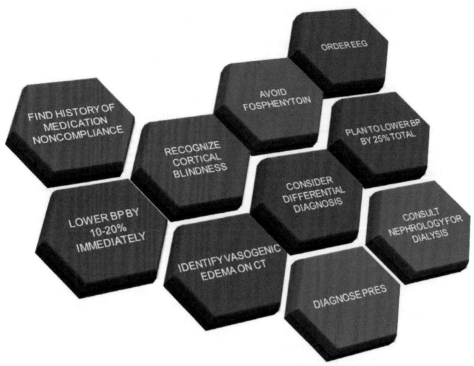

FIG. 16.1 Deconstructing key competencies in posterior reversible encephalopathy syndrome.

TABLE 16.2
Scenario Setup for Posterior Reversible Encephalopathy Syndrome

People needed	• Actor to play the patient • Actor to play ED nurse • Attending or Neurocritical Care Fellow to facilitate
Equipment needed	• Laboratory results • Syringes • Blood pressure cuff • IV access
Setup needed	• Monitor showing sinus rhythm, elevated blood pressure, and chest X-ray pulled up • Neuroimaging available (monitor turned off until imaging requested)

TABLE 16.3
Instructions to Actor Before Simulation

• Do not make eye contact with the learner; look just past them but in their general direction

• Try to avoid blinking with examiner approaching with hand

• Deny light when shown

• Normal language and speech

• Appear disoriented in time and place

• Wait for repeated instructions before performing a task

lorazepam and orders 30 mg/kg of IV valproate. He opts to avoid fosphenytoin because of its hemodynamic effects to prevent marked blood pressure lability. Synthesizing the presence of encephalopathy, cortical blindness, seizure, posterior predominant radiographic edema, and acute hypertension in the setting of renal failure, *L* diagnoses PRES, informs *CONF* that a lumbar puncture will not be necessary, and requests admission to the neurosciences intensive care unit with admission orders including EEG monitoring, nephrology consultation for hemodialysis, and titration of IV nicardipine (or another fast-acting, easily titratable infusion) to a target systolic BP of 190–210 mmHg. Scenario ends.

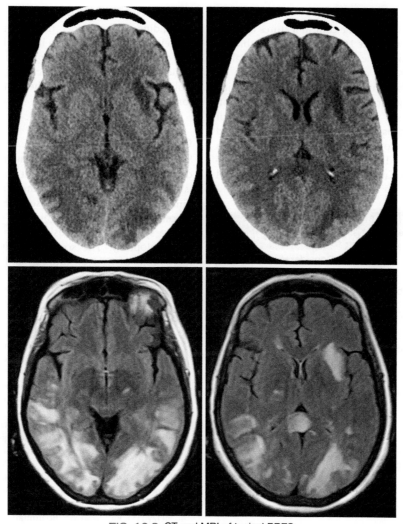

FIG. 16.2 CT and MRI of typical PRES.

THE NOT–SO–IDEAL LEARNER

There are many possible interventions and a high probability for error. The most commonly encountered misjudgments are listed below:

1. *The clinical presentation is considered secondary to encephalitis, systemic infection, or ischemic stroke.* It is expected that first-year residents or non-neurology fellows may miss the diagnosis, but cues will be provided by the confederate.
2. *The learner fails to use the appropriate antihypertensives.* The learner might use inappropriate antihypertensives (e.g., diuretics or long-acting agents such as enaprilat) or might continue to rely on bolus doses rather than moving to an infusion to improve control.
3. *The learner causes the blood pressure to drop precipitously.* The learner chooses a target blood pressure greater than 25% of the presenting pressure. This may lead to an abrupt reduction in the level of consciousness or prompt refractory seizures. Combining fosphenytoin loading with antihypertensives may lead to significant hypotension necessitating resuscitation for shock.
4. *The learner treats inadequately for hypertension.* The learner does not reduce blood pressure adequately, resulting in ongoing seizures and need for intubation.
5. *The learner does not diagnose the condition on CT or MRI.* This may prompt remediation.

DEBRIEFING

The debriefing can discuss the clinical features of PRES and its management. Table 16.4 shows the available antihypertensives, and in the debriefing, the pharmacological characteristics and dosing of these drugs can be reviewed. It is also important to discuss the specific goals and consequences of treatment. The condition should be discussed in full including its differential diagnosis, predisposing factors (Table 16.5), and well-described neuroimaging findings. The pitfalls in recognition can be discussed with a focus on misdiagnosis of cerebral infarcts rather than reversible cerebral edema.

TABLE 16.4
Drugs for Management of Hypertensive Crisis

Drug	Considerations
Labetalol • 10–20 mg IV bolus every 10 min • 0.5–2 mg/min IV infusion	• Hypotension • Bradycardia • Bronchoconstriction • Short-acting
Hydrazaline • 5–10 mg IV bolus	• Short-acting • Tachycardia • Worsening angina
Nicardipine • 5–15 mg/h IV infusion	• Significant hypotension • Rebound hypertension
Clevidipine • 1–2 mg/h IV • Maximal 20 mg/h	• Nausea • Dyslipidemia • Tachycardia • Very short half-life • Costly

TABLE 16.5
Predisposing Factors for Posterior Reversible Encephalopathy Syndrome[12]

Acute hypertension
Renal failure
Autoimmune disorders
Thrombotic thrombocytopenic purpura
Hemolytic uremic syndrome
Sepsis
Cytotoxic drugs (e.g., cyclosporine)

ADAPTING THE SCENARIO

Depending on the learner, the severity of hypertensive sequelae can be expanded to impending cardiac failure and development of pulmonary edema and hypoxemia. Abnormal troponins due to increased demand and diastolic failure can be added if the scenario is developed for emergency physicians.

CONCLUSIONS

Severe hypertension may present in the emergency department and requires urgent management. This is more pertinent in patients developing PRES. This scenario has been chosen because there is a perceived increase (and a number of missed cases) in the syndrome previously known as hypertensive encephalopathy. The scenario easily lends itself to discussions of CT scan findings and choosing hypertensive drugs.

REFERENCES

1. Whelton PK, Carey RM, Aronow WS, et al. 2017 ACC/AHA/AAPA/ABC/ACPM/AGS/APhA/ASH/ASPC/NMA/PCNA guideline for the prevention, detection, evaluation, and management of high blood pressure in adults: a report of the American College of Cardiology/American Heart Association Task Force on Clinical Practice Guidelines. *Hypertension.* 2018;71:e13–e115.
2. Fugate JE, Rabinstein AA. Posterior reversible encephalopathy syndrome: clinical and radiological manifestations, pathophysiology, and outstanding questions. *Lancet Neurol.* 2015;14:914–925.
3. Brady E, Parikh NS, Navi BB, et al. The imaging spectrum of posterior reversible encephalopathy syndrome: a pictorial review. *Clin Imaging.* 2018;47:80–89.
4. Hefzy HM, Bartynski WS, Boardman JF, et al. Hemorrhage in posterior reversible encephalopathy syndrome: imaging and clinical features. *AJNR Am J Neuroradiol.* 2009;30:1371–1379.
5. Bartynski WS, Boardman JF. Distinct imaging patterns and lesion distribution in posterior reversible encephalopathy syndrome. *AJNR Am J Neuroradiol.* 2007;28:1320–1327.
6. Covarrubias DJ, Luetmer PH, Campeau NG. Posterior reversible encephalopathy syndrome: prognostic utility of quantitative diffusion-weighted MR images. *AJNR Am J Neuroradiol.* 2002;23:1038–1048.
7. Karia SJ, Rykken JB, McKinney ZJ, et al. Utility and significance of gadolinium-based contrast enhancement in posterior reversible encephalopathy syndrome. *AJNR Am J Neuroradiol.* 2016;37:415–422.

8. Tong KA, Ashwal S, Holshouser BA, et al. Hemorrhagic shearing lesions in children and adolescents with posttraumatic diffuse axonal injury: improved detection and initial results. *Radiology.* 2003;227:332–339.

9. Ducros A. Reversible cerebral vasoconstriction syndrome. *Lancet Neurol.* 2012;11:906–917.

10. Datar S, Singh TD, Fugate JE, Mandrekar J, Rabinstein AA, Hocker S. Albuminocytologic dissociation in posterior reversible encephalopathy syndrome. *Mayo Clin Proc.* 2015;90(10):1366–1371.

11. Gao B, Lerner A, Law M. The clinical outcome of posterior reversible encephalopathy syndrome. *AJNR Am J Neuroradiol.* 2016;37:E55–E56.

12. Gao B, Lyu C, Lerner A, et al. Controversy of posterior reversible encephalopathy syndrome: what have we learnt in the last 20 years? *J Neurol Neurosurg Psychiatry.* 2018;89:14–20.

CHAPTER 17

Simulating Brain Death

Brain death occurs when a catastrophic acute brain injury leads to the irreversible cessation of all functions of the entire brain including the brainstem.[1] In the absence of dedicated neurointensivists or neurosurgeons in day-to-day practice, it is a burdensome task to ensure the competency of physicians to diagnose brain death. Simply said, it is a very-low-frequency event, and thus, experience is difficult to build. Moreover, because most patients do not progress to brain death and early examination may be unreliable due to sedation or alcohol intoxication, teaching situations that confound the examination of brain death become far more important than teaching how to run a series of neurologic tests.

Simulation of a brain death determination poses immediate problems. First, although a mannequin in current use can demonstrate abnormal vital signs, examination of brainstem reflexes cannot be completely done because most of these reflexes have not been built into these devices. Therefore, patients who do not yet fulfill the criteria of brain death—those with some reflexes spared—cannot be simulated with the notable exception of a patient with only a preserved breathing drive. Second, who should be taught—and thus by implication allowed—to perform such an examination— the neurologist, the neurosurgeon, the neurointensivist, the trauma surgeon, anesthesiologists with critical care training, or the general intensivist? Third, how do we train physicians to communicate compassionately with distraught (and sometimes visibly upset) family members confronted with the sudden death of a person still on a ventilator and receiving a significant level of support?

Experienced practitioners know that the diagnostic challenge in brain death determination is to eliminate all potential confounders and mimickers, and accomplishing this should be the specific focus of the simulation. Moreover, the systemic manifestations of brain death (i.e., diabetes insipidus, hypothermia, and hypotension) can be simulated, allowing learners to see the pattern firsthand and how to manage it. We have found it feasible to develop a skill set required to determine brain death through simulation and to show learners what is required to do a thorough diagnostic evaluation and how to recognize common pitfalls.[2,3]

THE PROBLEM BEFORE US

The clinical diagnosis of brain death medically determines a person's death.[1] As mentioned earlier, it is an uncommon neurologic state diagnosed in US tertiary medical centers in approximately two patients per month.[4] In the absence of major confounders, when all testable brainstem reflexes are absent and the patient is demonstrably apneic, no intervention and no amount of time can reverse the condition.[4] Along with absence of brainstem reflexes and apnea, patients typically have hypotension, hypothermia, and polyuria—if not already corrected.

Diagnosis is achieved by an organized, stepwise clinical examination adhering to published guidelines.[4] The process can be divided into three parts: (1) assessment of prerequisites, (2) examination, and (3) apnea testing. Step 1 establishes the cause of coma, confirms futility of intervention, and excludes confounders. Step 2 confirms the absence of brainstem reflexes and motor responses. Step 3 conclusively determines the absence of a respiratory drive.

The cause of coma is usually easily determined through the history, neuroimaging, or laboratory evaluation. After the clinical decision not to intervene further, some waiting period should follow to ensure no recovery. Neuroimaging should be consistent with coma. Traumatic brain injury remains the most common cause of coma leading to brain death.[5] The expected findings should include significant brain swelling, shift of the brainstem and other brain tissue (i.e., uncal or tonsillar herniation), intrinsic brainstem destruction, or, less commonly, diffuse cerebral edema with loss of sulci, and effacement of the cisterns due to anoxic-ischemic brain injury or exsanguination. The presence of sedative drugs and alcohol must be excluded through history and, often, toxicology screening. Drugs administered, often in the course of initial stabilization, could postpone the examination until 5 half-lives have passed assuming normal hepatic and renal function. If the patient had a major polytrauma or cardiopulmonary resuscitation for cardiac arrest, these organs may have become injured, prolonging clearance even more. The presence of severe acid base, electrolyte, or endocrine abnormalities may indicate an undetected ingested compound, and these should be excluded if feasible. The core body temperature must be normal or near normal (between 36 and 39°C) before the examination can begin. While very low temperatures are necessary to affect the brainstem reflexes, milder hypothermia may still alter the arterial pCO_2 rise sufficiently to affect apnea testing.[4] A forced-air warming blanket corrects hypothermia in most instances. Systolic blood pressure increased to $\geq$100 mmHg with fluids and vasoconstrictive agents will ensure reliability of the examination.

The ventilator should indicate absence of spontaneous, patient-triggered respirations when in a spontaneous breathing mode of ventilation. Autocycling, a phenomenon in which reduced airway pressure or flow triggers repetitive, "cyclical" ventilator-administered breaths, can be misinterpreted as spontaneous breathing by the patient.

The examination itself proceeds in normal fashion beginning with examination of pupillary reactivity to bright light, corneal reflexes, oculocephalic reflexes, oculovestibular reflexes, facial movement to noxious stimulus applied centrally at the supraorbital nerve or temporomandibular joint capsule, and motor response to noxious stimulus applied to each extremity. If all function is absent, the examiner proceeds to apnea testing.

Apnea-testing preparation involves preoxygenation with 100% oxygen for 15 minutes and ensuring that the patient does not desaturate with a positive end expiratory pressure (PEEP) of 5 cm H_2O. Apnea testing then proceeds with disconnection of the ventilator and delivery of 100% oxygen at 6 L/min via a tracheal-insufflation catheter guided to the level of the carina.[6] The chest should be uncovered. Observation of clavicular elevation, chest expansion, or abdominal excursion indicates breathing, which may only occur once during the testing period. After 8 minutes have passed, an arterial blood gas (ABG) is obtained. The patient is declared dead if no respirations have occurred and the arterial pCO_2 is $\geq$60 mmHg or 20 mmHg above the normal baseline. The normal baseline for a patient with obstructive lung disease is the pCO_2 at which they function optimally.

Ancillary (confirmatory) tests are not required in the United States but are performed when essential parts of the evaluation cannot be performed, usually when the apnea test is too complicated and unsafe in patients with chest trauma and poor lung function. A number of tests are available with variable sensitivity and specificity.[7]

Next, the diagnosis must be communicated to the next of kin. Following the declaration of death, the physician meets with family members and the room nurse and conveys the diagnosis of death in absolute terms. Normal reactions include grief, surprise, disbelief, or even anger, and these must be allowed; the physician should reassure the family that nothing could have changed the outcome. Some families may require further explanation of events. When appropriate, the physician then explains that the ventilator will be disconnected and medications stopped given that the person is dead and that the only reason to continue support would be possible organ donation. After the family conference, the organ procurement representative meets with family members to discuss organ donation.

THE PRESENTING CLINICAL PROBLEM

The patient is a 48-year-old man whose wife found him unresponsive in their yard near a ladder; apparently, he had been cleaning the gutters on his day off. She called 911, and paramedics arrived 15 min later and found no pulse. The monitor showed pulseless electrical activity (PEA). After 20 min of cardiopulmonary resuscitation and advanced cardiac life support, return of spontaneous circulation was achieved. The patient has been stabilized; given his initial PEA rhythm, he is not a candidate for targeted temperature management. CT scan of the brain shows severe, diffuse cerebral edema with absent sulci, intracranial hemorrhage in multiple compartments, effacement of the cisterns, and extensive skull base fractures. Neurosurgery evaluation found no brainstem reflexes and no operable lesions. The neurosurgery service informed the family that no intervention would benefit him. Two hours after the patient's arrival in the emergency department, the learner is asked to do a brain death examination. The patient's spouse has already been informed about the cardiac arrest and the suspicion of serious brain injury. The objectives are to (1) establish the history, (2) complete a brain death examination according to the established guidelines,[6] (3) effectively communicate the diagnosis of brain death to the patient's spouse, and (4) introduce the organ-procurement representative. The scenario has been deliberately initiated in the emergency department to emphasize it is not the place to proceed with a full examination; this should occur only after passage of more time and transfer of the patient to an intensive care unit. There is no room for mistakes; a quick assessment of brain death, even if requested, is poor practice and potentially erroneous. Key objectives and competencies are summarized in Table 17.1 and Fig. 17.1.

TABLE 17.1
Objectives

- Complete a brain death examination according to the 2010 AAN Guidelines[6]
- Improve knowledge of pitfalls in brain death evaluation
- Perform an adequate apnea test and understand physiology of the oxygen diffusion method
- Identify and correct major confounders
- Discuss appropriate use and limitations of ancillary tests used to support a clinical declaration of brain death
- Communicate a diagnosis of brain death with relatives

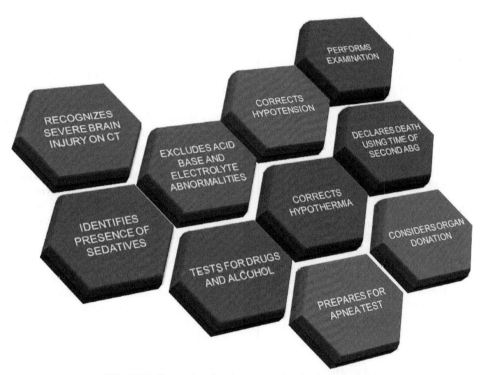

FIG. 17.1 Deconstructing key competencies in brain death.

Preparation

The mannequin is placed in a hospital bed in the ED, intubated, mechanically ventilated, a central venous catheter inserted, and vital signs showing on the monitor. The mannequin should show fixed, dilated pupils. Before the simulation, learners receive brain death guidelines to review in advance of the scenario.[6] Additional setup and equipment required are detailed in Table 17.2. The mannequin is ideally suited for the portrayal of brain death. It is immobile with eyes closed and pupils dilated and fixed to light. The jaw is slack and tone flaccid. Spinal reflexes cannot be simulated.

Coaching Actors

Instructions for actors (in this scenario, they only portray facilitators and family members) are shown in Table 17.3. Owing to the complexity of the subject, trained medical personnel are best suited for both the nurse and respiratory therapist roles. The confederate in this scenario is the nurse. The nurse answers the learner's questions and simulates the performance of actions as instructed by the learner. The respiratory therapist (RT) helps with assessment of cough and with apnea testing. This includes drawing ABGs from the arterial line and providing results to the learner as requested.

TABLE 17.2 Scenario Setup for Brain Death Examination	
People needed	<ul><li>Actor to play the nurse (registered nurse preferred)</li><li>Actor to play respiratory therapist (RT); respiratory therapist preferred</li><li>Actor to play the patient's spouse (layperson)</li><li>Attending or Neurocritical Care Fellow to facilitate</li></ul>
Equipment needed	<ul><li>Penlight</li><li>50 cc syringe</li><li>Empty pitcher to simulate "ice water" container</li><li>Box of tissue, Q-tips and saline bombs</li><li>Reflex hammer</li><li>Tracheal insufflation catheter</li><li>Mechanical ventilator</li><li>Laboratory results</li></ul>
Setup needed	<ul><li>ED Face Sheet in folder attached to the door</li><li>Monitor showing sinus rhythm and systolic blood pressure of 90 mmHg</li><li>Ventilator set to SIMV, rate 26, FiO2 40%, tidal volume 460 mL, pressure support 10, positive end expiratory pressure (PEEP) 15 cm H20</li><li>SimMan 3G on hospital bed endotracheally intubated with size 7.5 ETT secured/24 cm @ lip, pupils nonreactive, and blink shut off (eyes closed)</li><li>BP cuff, ECG leads, pulse oximetry, peripheral IV x2, IJ CVC, and arterial line attached</li><li>Catheterized with Foley catheter with CritiCore set to 33.5 C</li></ul>

The actor portraying the patient's spouse should be a layperson, who will more convincingly react to good or poor communication by the learner. The layperson is more likely to notice and question medical jargon. The "spouse" should question the learner's meaning until the learner clearly states with compassion that patient is dead ("not with us anymore" or "gone").

THE IDEAL LEARNER

L enters the room, introduces herself, and informs *CONF* that the patient should be admitted to the neurosciences intensive care unit (NICU) because he received sedating drugs for intubation (noted on the ED face sheet). She briefly examines *P*, testing level of consciousness, pupillary light reflexes, corneal reflexes, and motor response and finds them to be absent. She instructs *CONF* to place *P* in a cervical collar and orders a full set of labs. She looks at the monitor, noting the presence of a central line, low central venous pressure, hypotension, and hypothermia. She instructs *CONF* to give 1 L of lactated ringers, start a norepinephrine infusion to maintain the systolic BP ≥ 100 mmHg, and to place a Bair Hugger on the patient to warm him to $\geq 36°C$. *L* then reviews the previously ordered laboratory results. Finding an uncompensated respiratory alkalosis, normal drug screen, and no evidence of alcohol intoxication, she directs *CONF* to reduce the respiratory rate on the ventilator. *CONF* calls the respiratory therapist to carry out these instructions. Her attention now on the ventilator, *L* further instructs RT to reduce the positive-end expiratory pressure (PEEP) to 5 cm H_2O and monitor the oxygen saturation. She then asks to meet *P*'s spouse and is directed to an adjacent room where she is waiting.

L asks the spouse to explain what she has been told. *L* then confirms the irreversibility of the brain injury and

TABLE 17.3 Instructions to Actors Before Simulation
<ul><li>Mannequin-based scenario but also requiring actors to portray a respiratory therapist, nurse, and spouse</li><li>Nurse tells learner, "I've never seen this [brain death examination] performed in the ED before."</li><li>Respiratory therapist assists with full procedure of apnea testing (suction, alarms, changing ventilator settings, autocycling, use of insufflation catheter)</li><li>Spouse will ask questions about the procedure and ask if the patient will recover ("you always hear of people being in a coma for a long time and then having surprising recoveries")</li><li>If the learner uses the term "brain death," spouse asks "what is the difference between brain death and regular death" or states "but why is his heart still beating?"</li></ul>

states that *P* is in a coma. She further explains that if he does not improve, an extensive examination will be performed to test whether he has lost all brain function. She answers questions directly, correctly, and with compassion.

L returns to the room where *CONF* informs her that *P* is now in the NICU and that it is the following day. *L* inquires whether *P* has shown any signs of improvement and is informed there has been no change. *L* asks the respiratory therapist to increase the FiO2 to 100% and to switch the ventilator to a spontaneous mode. When the ventilator begins cycling at 14 breaths per minute on a spontaneous mode of ventilation, *L* expresses concern about autocycling and directs RT to return the ventilator to a controlled mode of ventilation.

L proceeds with a neurologic examination. When the absence of brainstem and motor responses is confirmed, she proceeds with apnea testing. *L* requests a new ABG and learns it is normal apart from a partial pressure of oxygen of 220. She instructs *CONF* to watch the monitor for the duration of apnea testing and to report vital signs aloud every minute. She uncovers *P*'s chest and instructs the respiratory therapist to disconnect the ventilator and provide oxygen at 6 L/min via a tracheal-insufflation catheter inserted to the level of the carina. She instructs the respiratory therapist to draw an ABG after 8 min and closely observes *P*'s chest, abdomen, neck, and shoulders. After 8 min (usually about 1 min of real time), *L* interprets the ABG as being consistent with brain death and declares death.

L reconnects the ventilator and asks to speak with *P*'s spouse. She clearly and compassionately tells the spouse that *P* is dead, answers her questions, and informs her that an organ-procurement representative will meet with her to discuss the possibility of organ donation. Scenario ends.

THE NOT-SO-IDEAL LEARNER

We have identified the following common missteps:

1. *Learner proceeds with examination in the ED.* Brain death examinations should not be performed in emergency departments. Time is required to clarify the history and ensure that all prerequisites have been met. Furthermore, the family needs this time to accept the fact that no treatment will help their loved one.
2. *Learner does not take time to confirm the history, ensure irreversibility, and review neuroimaging.* The neuro-imaging must explain the mechanism of coma. Uncertainties in the history should prompt extra caution.

3. *The learner does not consider sedative, analgesic, or paralytic drugs or assumes they have been adequately cleared.* The patient was previously intubated with succinylcholine, midazolam, and fentanyl. The half-life of midazolam and fentanyl is 6 h; the patient should be admitted and the examination delayed until 5 half-lives have passed. If the learner completes a brain death examination without first inquiring about sedating drugs, we deliver a breath to the mannequin during the apnea test.
4. *The learner does not consider illicit drugs, alcohol, or temperature.* The patient is a young man who fell from a roof on a day off, and alcohol or drugs must therefore be considered. Learners correct hypothermia when identified. More commonly and surprisingly, learners fail to ask about temperature at all.
5. *The learner is inadequately prepared for apnea testing.* Even when a checklist is provided, learners often fail to prepare for apnea testing. Common errors include omission of preoxygenation, transitioning directly from a high PEEP to ventilator disconnection, and omitting a baseline ABG pre-apnea testing after manipulating ventilator settings.

ADAPTING THE SCENARIO

This scenario is easily adaptable for different learners. Learners without a background in neurology (e.g., trauma surgery, anesthesiology, emergency medicine) benefit from having a checklist in hand.[4] However, providing a checklist to neurology and neurosurgery trainees is inadvisable because it eliminates the need for independent thinking. For neurocritical care fellows, the patient may have polyuria, hypernatremia, and more refractory shock requiring correction before performance of the examination. Learners may be capable of adjusting the ventilator settings to correct the acid base disorder. The introduction of ventilator autocycling increases the complexity of the scenario.

DEBRIEFING

The debriefing reviews, step by step (Fig. 17.2), the 25 assessments to declare a patient brain dead,[6] the appropriate indications for and limitations of ancillary tests used to support a clinical declaration of brain death, and tips for communicating with lay people about brain death and organ donation. The debriefing should focus on the recognition of confounders, and key competencies are emphasized. Any of the following missteps constitute automatic failure and require remediation: (1) failure to inquire about alcohol/drugs, (2) failure to recognize and correct hypothermia, (3) failure

25 Assessments to Declare a Patient Brain Dead

Prerequisites (ALL MUST BE CHECKED)

1. ☐ Coma, irreversible and cause known
2. ☐ Neuroimaging explains coma
3. ☐ Sedative drug effect absent
   (*if indicated, order a toxicology screen*)
4. ☐ No residual effect of paralytic drug
   (*if indicated, use peripheral nerve stimulator*)
5. ☐ Absence of severe acid-base, electrolyte, or endocrine abnormality
6. ☐ Normal or near normal temperature
   (*core temperature ≥ 36°C*)
7. ☐ Systolic blood pressure ≥ 100 mm Hg
8. ☐ No spontaneous respirations

Examination (ALL MUST BE CHECKED)

9. ☐ Pupils non-reactive to bright light
   (*typically mid-position at 5-7 mm*)
10. ☐ Corneal reflexes absent
    (*use both saline jet and tissue touch*)
11. ☐ Eyes immobile, oculocephalic reflexes absent (*tested only if C-spine integrity ensured*)
12. ☐ Oculovestibular reflexes absent
    (*50 cc of ice water in each ear sequentially*)
13. ☐ No facial movement to noxious stimuli at supraorbital nerve or temporo-mandibular joint compression.
    (*absent snout and rooting reflexes in neonates*)
14. ☐ Gag reflex absent (*gloved index finger to posterior pharynx*)
15. ☐ Cough reflex absent to tracheal suctioning (*at least 2 passes*)
16. ☐ No motor response to noxious stimuli in all 4 limbs (*triple flexion response is most common spinal-mediated reflex*)

Apnea Testing (ALL MUST BE CHECKED)

17. ☐ Patient is hemodynamically stable
    (*systolic blood pressure ≥ 100 mm Hg*)
18. ☐ Ventilator adjusted to normocapnia
    ($PaCO_2$ *35-45 mm Hg*)
19. ☐ Patient pre-oxygenated with 100% oxygen for 10 minutes ($PaO_2 ≥ 200$ *mm Hg*)
20. ☐ Patient maintains oxygenation with a PEEP of 5 cm H_2O (*if not, consider recruitment maneuver*)
21. ☐ Disconnect ventilator
22. ☐ Provide oxygen via an insufflation catheter to the level of the carina at 6 liters/min or attach T-piece with CPAP valve @ 10-20 cm H_2O and resuscitation bag
23. ☐ Spontaneous respirations absent
24. ☐ Arterial blood gas drawn at 8-10 minutes, patient reconnected to ventilator
25. ☐ $PaCO_2 ≥ 60$ mm Hg, or 20 mm Hg rise from normal baseline value
    or
    Apnea test aborted and confirmatory ancillary test (*EEG or cerebral blood flow study*)

Repeat Examinations

- Newborn (≥ 37 weeks gestational age) to 30 days: 2 examinations, 2 separate physicians, 24 hours apart
- 30 days to 18 years: 2 examinations, 2 separate physicians, 12 hours apart
- ≥18 years: 1 examination (*a second examination is needed in some U.S. states: AL, CA, FL, IA, KY, LA*)

Documentation

- Time of death (*use time of final blood gas result or use time of completion of ancillary test*)

FIG. 17.2 Check list to assist in examining a patient for brain death (used with permission of Mayo Foundation for Medical Education and Research).

to suggest admission to an ICU, and (4) performance of exam before drugs have cleared. Before remediation, learners view a video demonstrating the proper performance of the brain death examination.[8] The debriefing should also cover examination technique (e.g., how to test the gag reflex or ensuring a patent external auditory canal and visibility of the tympanic membrane before oculovestibular testing) and spinal reflexes. It is particularly effective to have the patient's "spouse" provide direct feedback to the learner. The facilitator should emphasize both the obligation of the physician to connect the family with the organ donation representative and the separation of the brain death diagnosis from transplant-related procedures.[5]

CONCLUSIONS

Through this pitfall-laden experience, learners develop an appreciation for the importance of organization and caution when determining brain death. Scenarios can be built to certify competence, but more importantly, learners must appreciate the complexity of evaluating a patient for possible loss of all brain function and subsequent organ donation.

REFERENCES

1. Uniform Determination of Death Act 12 Uniform Laws Annotated, in 589. 1993;(suppl 1997), West.
2. Hocker S, Schumacher D, Mandrekar J, et al. Testing confounders in brain death determination: a new simulation model. *Neurocrit Care.* 2015;23:401–408.
3. Wijdicks EF. Pitfalls and slip-ups in brain death determination. *Neurol Res.* 2013;35:169–173.
4. Wijdicks EF. *Brain Death.* 3rd ed. New York: Oxford University Press; 2017:296.
5. Nakamura MT, Rodio GE, Tchaicka C, et al. Predictors of organ donation among patients with brain death in the intensive care unit. *Transplant Proc.* 2018;50.
6. Wijdicks EF, Varelas PN, Gronseth GS, et al. Evidence-based guideline update: determining brain death in adults: report of the Quality Standards Subcommittee of the American Academy of Neurology. *Neurology.* 2010;74:1911–1918.
7. MacDonald D, Stewart-Perrin B, Shankar JJS. The role of neuroimaging in the determination of brain death. *J Neuroimaging.* 2018;28.
8. Wijdicks EF. Clinical diagnosis of brain death (video). In: *The Comatose Patient.* New York: Oxford University Press; 2014.

CHAPTER 18

Simulating Problematic Family Conferences

It has been said that the skill of communicating about disease and its consequences for our patients' lives is just as important as anything else we do in neurology. These (often very detailed) communications with those directly involved are best held in the form of a "family conference." For many intensivists, these meetings comprise a significant portion of overall care provided; therefore, counseling and guidance in family conferences should be included in a teaching curriculum.[1,2] It takes a considerable amount of time to update families (even more so when done poorly), and these conferences are difficult to schedule and even more difficult to complete because of interruptions (pagers going off or another patient in the unit becoming unstable). Similarly, teaching residents in the ICU is made more challenging because the considerable time commitment required conflicts with the competing demands of patient care.[3] In other words, the ICU is far from an ideal teaching environment for learning how to host these delicate discussions. Most communication teaching in any ICU consists almost solely of instructional videos, faculty observation, or a sit-down after an actual conference. Some research has been done in this area of communicating the patient's condition and prognosis. However, audio recording and playback of family conferences often highlight deficiencies in crucial domains (e.g., guidance, principles of shared decision-making, definition of futility, prognostication).[4]

A simulation center is perfectly suited to teach family conferences—unhurriedly—and can go beyond a "two-chair conversation" to offer a very realistic environment using a number of participants. Conducting a family conference for the main purpose of informing family members and discussing known or unknown patient wishes can be taught through role-playing.[5] Simulated family conferences can be structured, informative, and useful in teaching how to provide not-so-good news.

Multiple surveys and studies attest that families of very sick patients may overestimate the value of interventions, but on the other hand, physicians may undervalue interventions. Fortunately, in many cases—after an adequate explanation—common sense prevails,

and consensus between families and the healthcare team can be achieved. When the balance between benefits and harms becomes less delicate, decision-making becomes less complex. This chapter discusses the principles of conducting a family conference, demonstrates how such a meeting can lead to family agreement (or discord), and, finally, offers instruction in defusing arguments to arrive at a satisfactory resolution.

THE PROBLEM BEFORE US

Most family conferences are set up to discuss the appropriateness of the degree of intensive care provided and to disclose a prognosis when intervention seems not to help the patient. Maintaining support and treating major complications each time they arise will eventually allow any family to come to grips with the reality of it all. Physicians are not required to continue futile—perhaps easiest defined as "useless"—treatment in stable patients and are not required to continue or escalate treatment in a rapidly deteriorating terminally ill patient.

Futility in the Neuro ICU

The term futility closely relates to the anticipated outcome of the patient ("nothing more than a shadow of oneself") and may go beyond pathophysiology (a large but "technically" survivable brain hemorrhage) to include quality-of-life considerations. When the term "futility" is used, it has important connotations. Definitions of medical futility can easily become gobbledygook, and families may wish to continue care even if the likelihood of improvement is highly improbable (as long as continuing care does not harm the patient). Costs—although they may be astronomical—are often covered by Medicare or other insurance and thus are not a factor in most families' decisions. Some family members may feel that continuing care means giving their loved one the best they deserve.

Futility may be understood in terms of probability, such as treatments that have a zero probability of success, but family members may not want to see this as an absolute or may not believe it. Often palliative care services become involved if consensus cannot be achieved, but their success in reaching resolution while others could not is not guaranteed.

The quality of the information provided is decisive for many family members. Judgments about biological futility fall within specialized medical opinion but also comprise subjective factors such as tolerance of a major disability. Families may not be fully able to judge the long-term effects of a major neurologic injury, and explanations about quality of life should follow. The affected areas of the brain will not only determine weakness or paralysis but also aphasia, apraxia, amnesia, neglect, and other deficiencies in cognitive domains.

The Family Conference

A family conference in the Neuro ICU or in the Emergency Department for a patient with an acute, devastating neurologic injury differs from family conferences in other units for five reasons. First, the patient is rarely part of the conversation and only discussed in the third person by family members, physicians, and nurses. This is a highly unsatisfactory situation and differs from conversations in most other contexts. Even if the patient is able to converse, insight might be impacted considerably and answers may be off. Second, and the most critically important distinguishing feature, the family often must make spur-of-the-moment decisions. These include intubation, acute neurosurgical intervention such as a craniotomy or ventriculostomy placement, and procedures that invade brain structures

and thus must be considered differently than, for example, an exploratory laparotomy. Third, the patient's family is acutely flustered and overwhelmed by the situation; this differs from a chronic-disease scenario, where everyone in the family could "see it coming." One can only imagine how difficult these situations are, particularly if the patient is a younger family member who was fine in the morning and deeply comatose in the afternoon. Fourth, the outcome is more difficult to determine and involves questions such as "Will he be able to walk?", "Will he be able to talk, read, feed himself, go places?" Family members often will say, "if you can't be sure and he is in no distress, why not give him a chance?" Neurologic disability is difficult to describe, and it is even more difficult to know whether the patient can handle these deficits. Just as we would be under similar circumstances, the patient's family is notoriously unprepared for these situations, and the onus is on the experienced neurologist to explain what neurologic morbidity and disability entail. Fifth, family members often make quite important decisions on life and death (i.e., withdrawal of support) in situations that may still be fluid and not established. Often there is insufficient time to come to a reasoned and informed decision.

A family conference is typically held in a separate place and best at a table allowing everyone to take notes if needed (Fig. 18.1). All closely involved family members (and power of attorney), nursing staff, and attending physicians and fellows should be present. The presence of clergy cannot be overstated. The meeting starts with introducing each other.

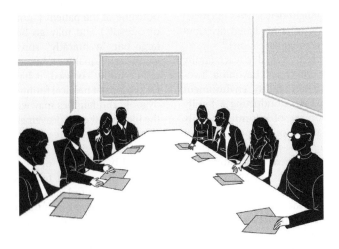

FIG. 18.1 Setup of family conference.

Conversations have to remain cordial and respectful. Attending physician starts with a summary of the neurologic condition and all interventions during the clinical course and may make use of neuroimaging to show the brain injury. The language used by physicians is very important and can be decisive in creating an environment of trust and shared decision-making or its opposite (i.e., conflict and distrust). The feelings cannot be normalized by empty phrases such as "Anyone would be confused by this situation" or "I understand what you are going through." Most families dread being confronted with feelings that can hardly be put into words.

Conflict between a family and physician can be defined as the inability to reach a consensus decision on the care of the patient. Physicians have appropriately shed the cloak of paternalism and have greatly improved in their ability to welcome family participation in the discussions and ultimate decision.[6] Generally, families make decisions for their loved one while trying to imagine how that individual would respond to a specific, severe disability. An advance directive can help— but not always because the language is often difficult to interpret. "If I become terminally ill, I do not want any heroic measures" is a common phrase in advance directives. These generic legal statements do confuse families and of course do not provide specific instructions to physicians. Physicians, thus, always have to translate the current medical assessment of the patient and interventions into what seems reasonable and what does not seem reasonable. For the neurologist, however, when caring for a patient who is absolutely dependent on others, doubly incontinent, fed by tube, and without any awareness of the environment or indication of responsivity, and no prospects of substantial improvement looking at the degree of injury, there is no question that we are witnessing a terminal state.

When families argue against futility (as defined by best medical knowledge), it creates a moral conflict and may seriously damage family-physician rapport. Simple attempts to persuade families to change course are counterproductive.[7] Moreover, language barriers may lead to poor communication ("lost in translation").[8] Family disagreements may result from differences of interpretation of presented information and facts, buried interpersonal feuds, and differences in the degree of the relationship with the patient. Religious preferences (with their often imposed limitations) seldom cause intrafamilial discord as families usually share the same beliefs. However, it can be a source of conflict if religious preferences differ within the family.

Major challenges to adequate family-to-physician communication remain, and there is no perfect answer. There is emerging evidence that proactive nurse participation improves dissemination of information and enhances trust.[9] Communication is best when it is symmetric (i.e., when all parties share equally in the discussion without one voice dominating and attempting to impose his or her will). We have seen that family conferences can be taught and structured. The main elements of a family conference are deconstructed in Fig. 18.2. The objectives of this scenario are shown in Table 18.1.

THE PRESENTING PROBLEM

In this simulation, the patient is a 74-year-old right-handed retired farmer with an acute left carotid artery occlusion resulting in an infarction of the middle cerebral artery and anterior cerebral artery territory. He is hemiparetic and globally aphasic. His level of consciousness is declining, and he needed intubation, which was performed a week before. His medical history is complicated by chronic lung disease, hypertension, and diabetes resulting in end-stage renal disease, and he is dependent on hemodialysis. Before this, he had lived at home but had difficulty remembering when to take his medication and required considerable help managing his affairs.

The main conflict presented here is that the son and daughter, both well-educated professionals, do not have the same opinion regarding the father's care. They both clearly do understand the outcome, recalling the father's friend who had a "bad stroke that left him disabled and in a nursing home." They are adamant that their father would not "want to end up like that." He always had a specific objection against being placed in a nursing home and definitely did not want to be on a mechanical ventilator for a prolonged period, nor did he want to continue dialysis in that state. He had often said, "A man should live at home or not at all." They both know what he would have wanted. However, while the son is willing to comply with the patient's wishes and favors strictly palliative care, the daughter favors taking a more proactive approach for their father because of a recent event that happened to one of her friends. This friend, who had a large stroke, is now home and only requires assistance with some activities of daily living. She is ambulatory and communicates although there is some difficulty. The daughter notes that the doctor predicted that her friend would never walk again, would be markedly disabled, and would need long-term nursing-home care. The prognosis in

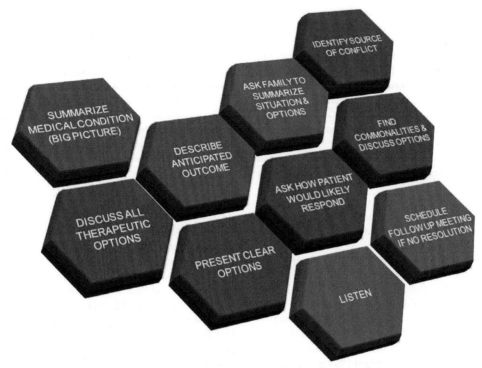

FIG. 18.2 Deconstructing key competencies in a family conference.

TABLE 18.1 Objectives
• To hold a successful family conference
• To identify and address a conflict
• To maintain trust in a setting of acrimony
• To defuse anger and redirect
• To practice negotiating consensus
• To involve all participants in the discussion
• To show genuine compassion
• To provide appropriate guidance and a recommendation if needed

TABLE 18.2 Scenario Setup for Family Conference		
People needed	1.	Actors to play son and daughter
	2.	Consider other family members
	3.	Facilitator
Equipment needed	1.	Conference room setup to mimic a comfortable waiting area
	2.	One-way mirror
	3.	Video-recording equipment
	4.	Box of tissue
	5.	Computer to show neuroimaging if appropriate

that case was completely wrong. The daughter argues that doctors are not so sure when it comes down to predicting the future—"not even the weatherman is good at it."

L is presented with an intrafamilial conflict in the absence of an advance directive. The options for the patient are fairly straightforward. One option is to let nature take its course; the other is to continue aggressive care. Both viewpoints are presented and, at some point,

may lead to a situation that may have periods of verbal abuse and anger. Both siblings seemed to have dug in their heels. The contribution of other family members is only confusing and not clear.

Preparation

It is important to stage the scenario in a large conference room with a number of attendees preferably sitting around a table (Table 18.2). The room should contain a one-way mirror to allow the facilitator to observe from a separate room, and the role-play should be videotaped for later debriefing. Tissues are on the table. Neuroimaging can be shown on an ipad. The participants include clergy, nursing staff, and residents. Each can be played by actors or invited residents. The conversation is largely between the daughter and son, who are the surrogate decision-makers, and the attending physician (in this case, L).

Coaching Actors

Most actors do not speak but may provide verbal cues by nodding or rolling their eyes. The scenario can be made more complicated by having the additional family members, residents and nurses offering their opinion, creating an initially uncontrollable conversation. This would allow L to focus the conversation and try to attend only to those family members who are decision-makers. The actors will be allowed time to develop their characters and will be allowed to improvise or rehearse or practice in the simulation center. For actors to carefully develop several stereotypical characters can be helpful (Chapter 3).

THE IDEAL LEARNER

The ideal learner would work through a set of important structured steps. In the best case scenario, L would start by discussing the big picture providing all relevant medical information and how the patient is experiencing this ordeal. He should adequately summarize the many underlying medical problems with some in an end-stage and the added effect of a major stroke. This is then followed by a discussion of current needs for ICU support and further potential therapeutic options. L would then ask how they want to proceed under these circumstances. L then progresses by explaining the expected outcome and briefly describing the disability outlook. L would also ask nursing staff and anyone else in the room to add to his assessment of the patient's problem. L would provide an environment of empathy, compassion, and trust. L would emphasize that shared decision-making is important. The conference largely focuses on trying to identify what the patient would want in that situation. L would then focus on how the opinions differ and continue to explain that family members are not denying their father a chance but that the outcome at his age and given his significant comorbidities is likely to be devastating. L would continue to emphasize hard clinical facts, findings on neuroimaging, and reiterate factual information. L should identify anxiety with family members and

try to provide comfort. L should identify the disagreement and summarize for all family members what the different positions are. L should emphasize that he does not want to deprive the patient of a possible good outcome but has to be fair in his assessment. Acknowledging to the daughter that physicians are not perfect prognosticators may help but it should be followed up why a good outcome is unlikely and what the criteria are for such a prognosis. In teaching institutions, decisions are rarely made by one person and many others have thought through this situation. L should explain in detail how comfort measures work and clarify that a change in the goals of care does not always result in early demise. The scenario does not require a resolution (or compromise)—which would be very unlikely after one family conference—but after this detailed conversation, the family should be well informed and allowed to rethink the matter. A subsequent conversation should be scheduled 24–48 h later, but the family is told that if they are ready to make a decision, a conference can be scheduled at any point in time.

THE NOT-SO-IDEAL LEARNER

We have noted that several important communication mistakes are possible, often as a result of not recognizing certain behaviors as summarized in Table 18.3. We can expect that learners will stray from what in

TABLE 18.3
Errors Noted During Family Conferences
• Poor structure
• Poor guidance
• Interrupting
• Failure to address disagreements
• Lack of empathy
• Rushed conversations
• Inconsistency
• Vagueness
• Too technical, use of medical jargon
• Uninformative
• Lack of closed loop communication
• No follow-up
• No decisions, just talk

essence is unknown turf for them. The most important missteps are summarized here.

1. *The learner is unable to provide a structure and guidance.* Failure to clarify a dispute may escalate the conflict. The learner does not recognize a conflict or its basis. The learner is unable to structure the conference to the essentials and to maintain control of the conversation.

2. *The learner fails to provide a clear explanation of the anticipated disability.* The learner has to try to summarize what neurologic disability entails and what type of help the patient would need in a nursing home. During these conversations, it is important to stick to the facts. Examples of miracle recoveries are often misjudgments, and many factors may play a role, often sedation. Without using too many technical explanations—actually showing what is normal brain on CT (all that is gray) and abnormal (all that is dark gray) may help families to understand the severity. This is preferable to giving a percentage ("40% of his brain is gone").

3. *The learner uses* platitudes or medical jargon. Phrases such as "you look sad," "I imagine this has been difficult," "I wish I had better news," or "anyone would be confused in this situation" may sound pleasant to family members, but do not effectively resolve the conflict. Moreover, it is important to offer clear explanations and not to overload the conversation with technical terms. These family conferences are also good practice opportunities to avoid empty words or other gestures that may not help and may, indeed, cause families to think the physician is insecure.

4. *The learner does not schedule a follow-up conference.* The conference ends with no clear decisions and further confusion on the part of family members. This is, of course, an undesirable outcome because the family conference has not produced any results.

5. *The learner does not defuse the tension.* The daughter will say "so you're just going to let my dad die?" or "so he will just starve to death" because the learner does not thoroughly explain the process of transition to comfort care and, in particular, that it involves treatments such as anxiolytics, anticholinergics, and opioids.

DEBRIEFING

The debriefing could use excerpts from the videotape that the facilitator identifies as potentially problematic. This can be done in the same session or at a later moment to allow the instructor to review the videotape

and choose excerpts to highlight. Again, debriefing should focus on relationship building with family members that emphasizes partnership and shared decision-making. The learner should be encouraged to describe their experience and whether he/she understood the conflict at hand.

During the debriefing, it is important to emphasize that the family is usually the best source for what the patient would have wanted and cares more about the patient's well-being than anyone else. It should be emphasized that families often find it difficult to live with the consequences of a decision. The debriefing should identify phrases that are not helpful but also point out elements of good communication used by the learner.

Debriefing of family conferences is far more time consuming if the learner wants to see the conversation replayed and to have error pointed out. One option is to collect a few taped conferences, save the common errors, and to discuss what the learner did well and what they could do better. Such an approach is a sensitive issue and appropriate care should be taken not to overcriticize.

A template for a successful family conference is shown in Table 18.4.

TABLE 18.4
Approach to the Family Conference

- Review the latest medical information.
- Have nursing staff present.
- Start by directing the focus to what the patient would want if he/she could understand the situation and speak for themselves
- Ask family members to summarize their understanding of the bigger picture.
- Gauge expectations (e.g., ask family members what would constitute futility in their minds and what an acceptable outcome would look like).
- Acknowledge the family's hope.
- Avoid defensive behavior.
- Maintain a lead and avoid discussions between small groups
- Acknowledge a willingness to be self-critical and understand that prediction is complex.
- Be flexible and acknowledge that the situation may change.

Adapted from Wijdicks EFM. *Communicating Prognosis.* New York: Oxford University Press; 2014.

CONCLUSION

The simulation of a family conflict in this setting between different family members is a common occurrence, and attending physicians caring for patients with acute neurological disease will have to know how to manage these situations. Several techniques are available, and enhanced role-playing is helpful to identify the empathy (or lack thereof) in a family that will come to bear in a family conference. Every element of a family conference can be scrutinized and tips or best practices can be provided. Experience over time has taught us behaviors to be avoided during family conferences. Not every conflict has to be resolved during the first meeting; keeping the lines of communication open is far more important. Families often recognize whom they can genuinely trust and whose approach is problematic.

REFERENCES

1. Curtis JR, Patrick DL, Shannon SE, et al. The family conference as a focus to improve communication about end-of-life care in the intensive care unit: opportunities for improvement. *Crit Care Med.* 2001;29:N26–N33.
2. Curtis JR, White DB. Practical guidance for evidence-based ICU family conferences. *Chest.* 2008;134:835–843.
3. Whitaker K, Kross EK, Hough CL, et al. A procedural approach to teaching residents to conduct intensive care unit family conferences. *J Palliat Med.* 2016;19: 1106–1109.
4. Cunningham TV, Scheunemann LP, Arnold RM, et al. How do clinicians prepare family members for the role of surrogate decision-maker? *J Med Ethics.* 2018;44:21–26.
5. Briggs D. Improving communication with families in the intensive care unit. *Nurs Stand.* 2017;32:41–48.
6. White DB, Braddock 3rd CH, Bereknyei S, et al. Toward shared decision making at the end of life in intensive care units: opportunities for improvement. *Arch Intern Med.* 2007;167:461–467.
7. Mehter HM, McCannon JB, Clark JA, et al. Physician approaches to conflict with families surrounding end-of-life decision-making in the intensive care unit. A qualitative study. *Ann Am Thorac Soc.* 2018;15:241–249.
8. Thornton JD, Pham K, Engelberg RA, et al. Families with limited English proficiency receive less information and support in interpreted intensive care unit family conferences. *Crit Care Med.* 2009;37:89–95.
9. Garrouste-Orgeas M, Max A, Lerin T, et al. Impact of proactive nurse participation in ICU family conferences: a mixed-method study. *Crit Care Med.* 2016;44:1116–1128.
10. Wijdicks EFM. *Communicating Prognosis.* New York: Oxford University Press; 2014.

Index

Note: Page numbers followed by "f" indicate figures and "t" indicate tables.

Printed and bound by CPI Group (UK) Ltd, Croydon, CR0 4YY

13/05/2025

01869735-0001